Sensory integrative
approaches in occupational...

Sensory Integrative Approaches in Occupational Therapy

Sensory Integrative Approaches in Occupational Therapy

Zoe Mailloux
Guest Editor

Occupational Therapy in Health Care
Volume 4, Number 2

The Haworth Press
New York

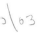
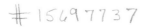

Sensory Integrative Approaches in Occupational Therapy has also been published as *Occupational Therapy in Health Care*, Volume 4, Number 2, Summer 1987.

The Haworth Press, Inc. 10 Alice Street, Binghamton, NY 13904-1580
EUROSPAN/Haworth, 3 Henrietta Street, London WC2E 8LU England

Library of Congress Cataloging-in-Publication Data

Sensory integrative approaches in occupational therapy.

"Has also been published as Occupational therapy in health care, volume 4, number 2, summer 1987" — T.p. verso.
    Includes bibliographies.
    1. Occupational therapy. 2. Sensory-motor integration. I. Mailloux, Zoe. [DNLM: 1. Occupational Therapy. 2. Perceptual Disorders — rehabilitation. 3. Psychomotor Disorders — rehabilitation. 4. Sensation — physiology.
W1 OC601H v.4 no.2 / WL 700 S4287]
RM735.S52   1987   615.8'5152   87-2878
ISBN 0-86656-665-1

Dedication

This issue is dedicated to A. Jean Ayres, PhD, OTR, FAOTA, in appreciation for the ways in which she has inspired countless occupational therapists in their professional pursuits.

Sensory Integrative Approaches in Occupational Therapy

Occupational Therapy in Health Care
Volume 4, Number 2

CONTENTS

FROM THE EDITOR'S DESK

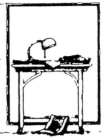

We are pleased to present to you in this issue what no doubt is the first, to our knowledge, of many collections of practice oriented papers on sensory integrative applications in occupational therapy. No topic seems to have aroused more widespread interest and curiosity than this now broadly applied theory originated by A. Jean Ayres. Therefore, it is fitting that the guest editor, Zoe Mailloux, who has known and worked with Jean over many years and is now the clinical and administrative director of the Ayres Clinic, in Torrance, California, has dedicated the issue to her. It is little enough to acknowledge in this way one who has had such a profound impact on occupational therapy practice and research.

I am much indebted to Zoe for her enlightened and creative design of the issue, for her resourcefulness in tapping some of the key practitioners of sensory integration principles across the spectrum of treatment problems which occupational therapists face. Yet these papers simply tap the potential. While the work of Ayres has been traditionally identified with early school age children, research is beginning to show that the principles of sensory integration have far wider applicability, as this issue attests. But the limits of this volume require that papers on work with neonates, with patients with disability from stroke, with broader applications to the aged, with chronic adult schizophrenia, and on how the therapist knows to select SI theory, as opposed to other commonly used neurobehavioral theories for a particular case, had to be saved for another time.

Especially welcome are the authors who have gone the extra step to show how sensory integration theory complements and finds mutual reinforcement with other common occupational therapy theory bases . . . in particular occupational behavior and the role theory, play behavior and adaptation that it encompasses. The closer we come as a profession to embracing a common, all-encompassing base framework for our very diverse practice, the closer we shall come to being a solid profession.

When I envisioned this issue, some 12-15 months ago, I had the advantage of being in Southern California where many advocates of sensory integration live and practice. Thus I had many advisors about content and possible editors and authors. I needed a guest editor to be sure, since I personally am far removed from most of current practice, and have never practiced with SI principles. I was led to Zoe Mailloux, and the issue's content attests to the rightness of that choice. But being a Southern Californian I could also not escape the exposure to the always exciting potentials of this theory and its application. One of those who has been responsible for my orientation and steady growth about the potentials of interest in sensory integration as a unifying concept in human development is Lawrene Barker Kovalenko. Lawrene's confidence in the concepts and in Jean Ayres' brilliance in developing the theory for occupational therapy practice led to the development of the CSSID (Center for the Study of Sensory Integrative Dysfunction), now SII (Sensory Integration International). The change in titles alone for that vigorous research organization testifies to the truth of her confidence. So, in a sense, the idea for this issue came also from Lawrene. And I thank her.

Along with the papers chosen for inclusion for the theme content of this issue comes Practice Watch, a usual feature of some timely practice topic, as well as a rich collection of reviews of current publications of interest to therapists.

Two forthcoming issues in this volume give equal promise of meeting popular practitioner, student and educator demand. One will be entitled: *The Occupational Therapy Manager's Survival Handbook,* and will contain in *case format* presentations and solutions to some of the persistent problems of administrators at all levels. Volume IV will close with *Hand Rehabilitation in Occupa-*

tional Therapy, a collection intended to supplement the resources available to therapists who deal with patients with hand problems within the context of a general, hospital practice but largely written by therapists who consider themselves hand "specialists." Watch for both of these important additions to occupational therapy libraries.

Florence S. Cromwell
Editor

Introduction

Zoe Mailloux, MA, OTR

Guest Editor

The concepts underlying sensory integrative theory and its application to patients with neurologic dysfunction were first proposed in the occupational therapy literature by Ayres during the late 1950's and early 1960's.[1-4] With roots in neurobiology, sensory integrative theory has evolved and expanded during the last several decades to become one of the more developed and sophisticated theoretical frameworks to emerge as an occupational therapy knowledge base.

The term sensory integration has been defined as ''the organization of sensory input for use.''[5,p.184] As a general concept, this term is applicable to the normal development of all sensory systems and their interrelated functions. Within the neurobiology literature, the term sensory integration is utilized to describe these processes in human and animal systems.[6] In developing sensory integrative theory from an occupational therapy perspective, Ayres has applied these neurobiological concepts to the capacity to learn, to organize behavior and to respond adaptively to the environment.[5]

As a continually developing and evolving theoretical perspective, sensory integration has produced identifiable principles and postulates which have helped to guide evaluation and treatment of certain disorders. However, comprehensive reviews of sensory integrative theory have differentiated this approach from others aimed as specific training or skill development often termed sensorimotor approaches and/or perceptual motor programs.[7,8] Differentiation of theoretical perspectives and critical analysis of how constructs can be appropriately combined in treatment is essential to the practicing therapist. Consideration of the ways in which theories might be applied to new or different problems is also important to the clinician.

Zoe Mailloux is Clinical Director at the Ayres Clinic, Torrance, CA.

5

The purpose of this special issue on sensory integration is, therefore, twofold. The first is to promote continued development of sensory integrative theory by examining differentiation as well as potential synthesis of this approach with concepts and practices of other frameworks. Secondly, this issue aims to provide examples of appropriate application of sensory integrative concepts to new or different aspects of occupational therapy.

In moving beyond the traditional application of sensory integrative theory with the elementary school aged child with learning disabilities, the papers in this issue consider the ways in which concepts from this theoretical framework might be applied to programs for infants, preschoolers, adolescents and the elderly. Authors with a wide array of clinical, research and education experience have addressed contemporary issues such as advocacy, cost effectiveness, family participation, documentation of patient progress school programming and computer application as well.

It is hoped that this collection of papers will become one of many such efforts aimed at expanding the work originally proposed by A. Jean Ayres. Therefore, the intent of this issue is to stimulate thinking and raise new questions which will promote continued development of sensory integrative theory as a vital component of occupational therapy in health care.

REFERENCES

1. Ayres, A.J.: The visual motor function. *Amer J. Occup Ther 12(3)*: 130-138, 1958

2. Ayres, A.J.: Development of body scheme in children. *Amer J Occup Ther (15)3:* 99-102, 1961

3. Ayres, A.J.: The Eleanor Clark Slagle Lecture, The development of perceptual-motor abilities: A theoretical basis for treatment of dysfunction. *Amer J Occup Ther (17)6:* 221-225, 1963

4. Ayres, A.J.: Tactile functions: Their relation to hyperactive and perceptual motor behavior. *Amer J Occup Ther (18)1:* 6-11, 1964

5. Ayres, A.J.: *Sensory Integration and the Child*, Los Angeles, CA: Western Psychological Services, 1979

6. Masterson, R.B. (Ed.): *Handbook of Behavioral Neurobiology, Vol. 1: Sensory Integration*, New York, Plenum Press, 1978

7. Clark, F., Mailloux, Z., and Parham, D.: Sensory integration and learning disabilities. In Clark, P.N. and Allen, A.S.: *Occupational Therapy for Children*, St. Louis, C.V. Mosby, 1985

8. Ottenbacher, K: Sensory integration therapy: Affect or effect. *Amer J Occup Ther 36(9):* 571-578, 1982

Appreciation is extended also to the following individuals who served as expert reviewers for this issue:

Barbara Burris, MHS, OTR

Terri Chew, MA, OTR

Florence Clark, PhD, OTR

Terri Crowe, MS, OTR

Susan Knox, MA, OTR

Lucy Miller, PhD, OTR

Diane Parham, MA, OTR

Gretchen Reeves, MA, MOT, OTR

Ruth Zemke, PhD, OTR

Maternal Role Preparation:
A Program Using Sensory Integration, Infant-Mother Attachment, and Occupational Behavior Perspectives

Janice Posatery Burke, MA, OTR, FAOTA
Florence Clark, PhD, OTR, FAOTA
Carol Hamilton-Dodd, MA, OTR
Toni Kawamoto, OTR

SUMMARY. The Maternal Role Preparation (MRP) project demonstrates an innovative occupational therapy approach to increasing maternal competence in first time mothers. This four session program provided women with discussion, demonstration, practice and written materials covering topics concerning their infants (attachment, sensory systems, developmental abilities) and themselves (acquiring a new role as mother). Theoretical constructs from Behavioral Pediatrics, Sensory Integration and Occupational Behavior were evaluated for their compatibility and combined under the unifying framework of Occupational Behavior. The program represents an opportunity for occupational therapists to combine sensory integration theory and practice with other compatible treatment perspectives and approaches.

. . . understanding of what is going on in her infant can reinforce a mother's best judgement and instincts, and above all, add to her pleasure. When parents enjoy interacting with their

Janice Posatery Burke is Adjunct Assistant Professor, Department of Occupational Therapy, University of Southern California and Private Practitioner, Culver City, California. Florence Clark is Associate Professor, Department of Occupational Therapy, University of Southern California. Carol Hamilton-Dodd is Occupational Therapist, Community Medical Center, Covina, California. Toni Kawamoto is Clinical Educational Specialist, Sepulveda Veterans Administration Hospital, Sepulveda, California.
This article appears jointly in *Sensory Integrative Approaches in Occupational Therapy* (The Haworth Press, Inc., 1987) and *Occupational Therapy in Health Care*, Volume 4, Number 2 (Summer 1987).

new baby, he in turn, becomes more rewarding. This circular process can only add luster to each of the participants.[1,p.36]

The maternal role preparation (MRP) program was designed to help first time mothers as they prepare for the birth of their child. Unlike traditional birth preparation classes which focus on learning physical and mental skills for labor and delivery of the infant, this occupational therapy program was developed to address a broad array of maternal skills that would be needed starting from the time of birth and extending into the newborn period.

In American society today, many young women have never been exposed to the caretaking of children before the birth of their own infant.[2] The decline of the extended family, more emphasis on early career development and delay in childbearing are among the reasons for this limited experience.[3] Women who have not had opportunities to learn about the early abilities of infants, how to effectively interact with them or how to manage the everyday demands of mothering may be "at risk" for developing feelings such as dissatisfaction and incompetence in their role as mother.

Maternal competence and adaptation has been observed and documented in contemporary research.[2,4] These factors are summarized in Table I. The variables found to be associated with successful mothering fall into two main categories. The first category is infant-mother attachment. This includes issues such as infant mother bonding, infant mother interaction and infant temperament. The second

TABLE I

FACTORS ASSOCIATED WITH SUCCESSFUL ENACTMENT OF

MOTHERING ROLE

Infant-Mother Bonding

Reciprocal Mother-Infant Interactions

Responsiveness of Infant to Mother

Maternal Perception of Infant

Provision of Appropriate Stimulation

to Infant

Understanding Infant's Temperament

Social/Emotional Support

category includes understanding the infant's abilities, individual differences, sensory systems and techniques for soothing and calming.

Parenting programs addressing infant-parent attachment have been implemented and have demonstrated success in fostering those interactions.[5] The intent of this project was to go beyond these areas of preparation to include a wider range of skills and habit patterns that would be needed by the woman entering her role as mother. In addition to infant-mother interaction skills, mothers would be taught stimulation techniques for their newborns and role skills including time and stress management, energy conservation and effective daily routine management. Although the fathering role is equally important and may require preparation, this program focuses on mothering as an initial step in developing this type of parenting program.

SELECTING A FRAMEWORK
AND DESIGNING A PROGRAM

> . . . therapists must draw from many knowledge sources to produce strategies for addressing the problems of the individual . . . [6,p.282]

Clinical practice in occupational therapy has become more complex as therapists address a larger scope of problem areas related to a person's everyday competence. With each new clinical puzzle "the therapist addresses the spectrum of behaviors that must function together to permit the individual to experience successful adjustment or adaptation to task and role demands."[6,p.290]

Effective programming is a result of thorough analysis of the problem and recognition of all possible treatment strategies. In many situations therapists may want to combine theories which define various aspects of the problem at hand.[7]

In this program the objective was to create opportunities for women to practice competent and efficacious behavior for their new roles, develop skills and habits that would support their new roles, as well as meet defined social requirements and provide meaning and satisfaction in their daily life routines. Program content was determined in two phases. The first included a literature review of historical and contemporary writings addressing mothers and infants, the second phase consisted of a "pilot study" including indepth interviews with new mothers for the purpose of identifying and/or clarifying program content.

In order to construct a program that would address infant-mother attachment, the sensory and developmental concerns in infancy and the skills to support effective role behavior in the mother, information from three distinct knowledge bases would have to be combined. The selection process included importing information from a field outside but closely related to occupational therapy and combining two theory bases already existing within the field. First, from the behavioral pediatric literature concepts regarding the critical importance of the infant-mother relationship, infant temperament, maternal perception of the infant and maternal-infant bonding were chosen as relevant and appropriate to the program intent. Second, from sensory integration theory the constructs concerning complex sensory systems of the infant and their need to be stimulated, soothed and reacted to were considered critical to the program. Third, the notions of role and role transition from occupational behavior were considered essential to successful facilitation of the mothering role (see Table II).

Additionally, because of the complexity of the behaviors being addressed, occupational behavior was selected as a conceptual framework for organizing the interdisciplinary constructs into a cohesive model. The occupational behavior perspective simultaneously looks at individuals and their environments. It accounts for the internal factors and external forces that direct a person's behavior. Governed by the laws of general systems theory (GST), this perspective provides a grounding for explaining the complex interactions of everyday life (such as performance, satisfaction, habits and change over time) with equal consideration given to related concepts.[8] Using the occupational behavior perspective, the program developers were able to simultaneously consider all of the behaviors deemed relevant to maternal role preparation.

PROGRAM DESCRIPTION

The Maternal Role Preparation program was initially developed as a research study designed to probe issues about maternal competence.[9,10] The study sought information in three areas: the combined sensory integration, infant-mother attachment and occupational behavior approach to programming and the association of the programming to maternal competence in maternal care behaviors; the

TABLE II

THEORY BASE	CONCEPTS
Sensory Integration	Infant Development
	Individual Differences
	Sensory Systems
	Infant Abilities at Birth
	Soothing & Calming Techniques
Occupational Behavior	Role Transition
	Skills & Habits for
	Role Enactment
	Biologic Needs of Mother
	-Exercise
	-Physiologic Changes
	Post Partum
	-Energy Conservation
	-Body Mechanics
Behavioral Pediatrics	Infant Mother Relationship
	Infant Mother Bonding &
	Attachment
	Infant Temperament
	Infant Development

self perceived adaptation of the woman to the maternal role; and whether participation in the program would be associated with satisfaction with maternal role preparation provided along with routine obstetric care. Factors considered beyond the scope of this pilot study included: paternal preparation, cultural and religious beliefs, socio-economic status, prior experience with children, desire to have children and parental treatment as child.

The program was divided into four sessions beginning before the birth of the baby (approximately one month) and ending when the baby was 2-3 weeks old. Each session followed an outline of goals derived from the guiding theoretical constructs and utilized discussion, prepared handouts and demonstration to teach information and facilitate skill acquisition (see Tables III, IV, V, VI). The mother was seen in her home for the first, third and fourth sessions. The second session was held in the hospital following the birth of the child. Each appointment was 1-2 hours in length with ample time allotted for discussing special concerns of the mother. Therapists were also available by telephone between appointments to answer questions and concerns.

FROM THEORY TO PROGRAM CONTENT

Infant-Mother Attachment

Maternal-infant bonding is an initial factor in establishing maternal sensitivity and understanding for her infant's need. This initial

TABLE III

TREATMENT SESSION 1

Place: Mother's Home
Duration: 1 hour
Target Date: Within 1 month prior to due date

Goals: 1. To develop rapport between therapist and mother.
2. To get a general impression of mother-to-be's concerns for the postpartum period.
3. To begin discussing alternatives for feeding the baby.

Methods: a. Discuss goals of the program and map out tentative schedule for the remainder of the program.
b. Discuss goals and interests of mother in general.
c. Open discussion about mother's general concerns during postpartum period and for caring for new infant.
d. Discussion on alternatives for feeding baby.
e. Direct mother to additional resources for support and information such as books, support groups and magazines.

Materials: Outline of program, calendar, bibliography of parenting books

TABLE IV

TREATMENT SESSION 2

Place: Hospital
Duration: 1 hour
Target Date: 1-2 days after the birth

Goals: 1. To provide the mother with information and handouts
           re: physiological changes in women postpartum.

        2. To provide the mother with information on breastfeeding
           and opportunity to practice breastfeeding techniques
           (only if mother chooses breastfeeding).

Methods: a. Discussion of physiological changes, resumption of
            normal cycles and importance of rest.

         b. Discussion of mother's concerns about physical and bodily
            changes and emotional feelings.

         c. Review of early postpartum exercises for mother.

         d. Discussion and opportunity for mother to practice
            breastfeeding and handling of infant.

         e. Explanation of Parent-Infant Care Record to be completed
            in following week.

Materials: Handouts: Breastfeeding myths and suggestions, Early
           postpartum exercises, Parent-Infant Care Record

process provides an important foundation or start point for attachment and the long term interaction process that follows. Developing maternal-infant interaction requires reading and reacting to reciprocal signals as part of a communication system. The mother's ability to read these signals and adapt her behavior according to the information she receives will lead to an increasingly responsive infant-mother relationship. The MRP program is designed to develop skills for such a relationship.

How a mother perceives her infant will influence her interaction with the infant and the type of environment she creates for the infant.[9] In the MRP program, mothers were given information that considered the child's temperament, her own feelings of compatibility with it and strategies for adapting care routines that would best match mother, infant and environment. In general, infants who were more irritable required more skill in handling and their mothers needed more assistance in learning these skills.

In addition to this basic information on the significance of an infant-mother relationship and the kind of factors that influence it positively and negatively, mothers were given opportunities to observe a therapist interacting with their infants and then modelled those behaviors and strategies with the babies. These demonstrations and materials dovetailed when shared with the sensory and developmental components of the program. The MRP program provided situations for mothers to learn about and become skillful in infant stimulation and play activities. These activities were viewed as interactions that promoted attachment between the mother and infant.

Sensory Characteristics of the Infant

The infant is constantly receiving and reacting to stimuli. [1,p.24]

Young infants are believed to be capable of effective interaction with the world around them. [11] In part, such interaction is based on the infants' sensory capabilities. It is also based on maternal percep-

TABLE V

TREATMENT SESSION 3

Place: Mother's home
Duration: 1 1/2 hours
Target date: 1 week after the birth

Goals: 1. To develop and organize a plan to help
              mother plan her day, conserve energy and
              use her time efficiently.

           2. To review and practice energy conservation
              techniques, body mechanics and postpartum
              exercises for the mother.

Methods: a. Discuss the Parent-Infant Care Record and
            time management.

         b. Discuss problems the mother may be having
            in organizing her day.

         c. Discuss energy conservation techniques.

         d. Discuss and practice body mechanic techniques
            and postpartum exercises.

         e. Discuss leisure activities and interests and
            feasibility of incorporating into daily life.

         f. Discuss mother's concerns and questions.

Materials: Map of a tentative daily schedule
            Handouts: Energy conservation, body mechanics,
            postpartum exercises for mother.

TABLE VI

TREATMENT SESSION 4

Place: Mother's home
Duration: 1-2 hours
Target Date: 2-3 weeks after the birth

Goals: 1. To foster the infant-mother relationship.

2. To provide the mother with information on various topics of infancy and to provide her with chance to practice handling and stimulating her baby.

Methods: a. Discuss early infant development and individual differences (reflexes, sleep patterns, infant temperament).

b. Demonstration and opportunity for mother to elicit reflexes and infant responses.

c. Discuss mother's feelings about her infant's temperament.

d. Discuss and demonstrate the infant's sensory systems and provide an opportunity for mother to practice infant stimulation activities.

e. Discuss suggestions for the mother to alter the environment to fit both infant's and mother's needs.

f. Discussion and practice of some exercises for mother and baby.

Materials: Handouts: Activities for infant stimulation, Age appropriate toys, Ideas for toys mother can make, Mother-baby exercises

tion of the baby's behavior, by beliefs the mother has about them and by her sensitivity and desire to respond to the baby's signals.[12]

Research in early infant behavior has revealed the sophistication and complexity of the sensory processing of the newborn. Touch, gravity and movement, muscle and joint sensations, sight, sound, smell and taste are all present in varying degrees of organization at birth. By one month of age infants are performing adaptive responses to sensation, many of which are built in at birth. The sensory integration that occurs in this sample sensory-motor activity of the infant provides a spring board for continued development given otherwise normal factors.[13] Mothers in the MRP program were given opportunities to understand the relationship between behavior they saw in their newborns and the children's long term growth and development.

The MRP program provided mothers with information on the developmental progressions that are typical in infancy. Discussions highlighted the uniqueness of an infant's sensory systems and appropriate stimulation techniques. Through demonstration and practice opportunities women were able to develop an understanding of their baby's needs and how those needs are communicated and manifested in the temperament, sleep wake cycles and play preferences of the infant. Newborns show a capacity to react differentially to stimulation and in fact will react positively to stimuli appropriate to him/her and turn away from stimuli that is negatively perceived.[1] These early sensory experiences are gradually organized within the brain and given new meaning as the child learns to focus attention on particular sensations and to ignore others.[13]

Mothers were taught cues that an infant gives regarding physical and emotional needs. Soothing and calming techniques were introduced along with sensory stimulating activities providing mothers with a repertoire of handling, caring and stimulating strategies. These early experiences in learning the most effective means of communication with the child and feeling effective in the communication process are early experiences that lay a foundation for a long term mother infant relationship.[12]

The Mothering Role

> The physical adjustment that a new mother is making after delivery lasts for many weeks. It is a strain on her resources both physical and emotional. It is largely responsible for her inability to sleep well, to eat properly, to keep her emotions in control.[1]

The occupational behavior perspective views habits and skills as components of role. It is the presence and incorporation of knowledge and skills into habits that support a person as they seek to fulfill the daily tasks of a given role. Generalized habits serve to form routines for behavior so that attention is directed only toward novel demands for skills. As new skills are acquired, skills are integrated into the habit structure.[14]

The transition process into a new role represents a crisis point for an individual. This is a time when a person needs opportunities to learn about their new role and develop skills in a supported situation. In this way the person has a chance to ask questions, clarify information and practice skills in a relatively safe environment with greater chance of later success in a less protected situation. Programs that offer "practice" simulations are designed to decrease vulnerability to failure. Recognizing the "at risk" situation of the woman entering her new role, allowed the program therapists to provide strategies and opportunities to practice and prepare for future task demands. In a general sense, the ease that individuals find in acquiring new roles is dependent upon their own adaptive nature. That ability to amend or elaborate on the skills they have and to make additions to their everyday habit structure requires flexibility, confidence and in many cases guidance and support.

Program content within the occupational behavior theory base included: physical and biologic changes of the mother, daily living activity exploration, stress and time management skill development. Knowledge of the physical changes that are undergone during the postpartum period is likely to contribute to better physical recovery and emotional adjustment. The MRP program provided information about major postpartum issues including fatigue, weight loss and physical exercise after childbirth and "baby blues."

Before the baby's delivery, the therapist and mother discussed the benefits of organizing customary daily activities allowing appropriate time for rest. Strategies for approaching the initial postpartum period included preplanning for arrangement of the home setting to maximally promote efficient child care and energy conservation, securing housekeeping and other support services, enlisting support systems available through family and friends, selecting diaper preference and insuring availability, and preparation and freezing of meals to sustain the family during the initial period after baby's birth. Following the birth, women who expressed interest in promoting weight loss and recovering muscle tone were shown an exercise plan. Initiation of the plan was subject to physician approval.

Possible psychological effects of hormonal changes that may occur after birth were discussed with all new mothers including differences in breastfeeding and bottle feeding women. This content was considered essential to mothers who would need to anticipate hormonal changes. The choice of whether a mother would breast or bottle feed was presented as an option to be handled by mother, her mate and the attending physician. Participants learned about postpartum blues and the characteristics of depression, despondency and weeping that are experienced in about two-thirds of all new mothers.[15] Being informed that this is a normal occurrence was considered important for mothers who would be faced with such feelings.

Through discussion and demonstration, mothers were exposed to work simplification techniques and organizational strategies for managing activities of daily living and facilitate efficient and economic work activity. Energy conservation techniques and body mechanics were also provided within the occupational behavior perspective.

SUMMARY

This Maternal Role Preparation program represents an innovative model of program development and service delivery for occupational therapy. In an effort to meet the complex needs of first time mothers, the program combined constructs from behavioral pediatrics, sensory integration and occupational behavior.

Four treatment programs were developed to address infant-mother attachment issues, the sensory, developmental and calming needs of the infant and the role transition challenges of the mother. Intervention approaches derived from these three compatible theories were translated into discussion, demonstration and practice situations and handout materials.

REFERENCES

1. Brazelton TB: *Infants and Mothers*. New York: Delacorte Press, 1969
2. Klaus MH, Kennell JH: *Parent-infant bonding* [2nd edition] St. Louis: CV Mosby Co, 1982
3. Brazelton TB, Als H: Four early stages in the development of mother-infant interaction. *Psychoanalytic Study of the Child* 34:349-369, 1979
4. Majewski JL: Conflicts, satisfactions, and attitudes during transition to the maternal role. *Nurs Res* 35: 10-14, 1986
5. Myers BJ: Early intervention using Brazelton training with middle-class mothers and fathers of newborns. *Child Development* 23: 329-334, 1982
6. Mailloux Z, Mack W, Cooper C: Knowing what to do: the organization of knowledge for clinical practice. In *Health Through Occupation*, G Kielhofner, Editor. Philadelphia: FA Davis Company, 1983
7. Burke JP: Defining occupation: importing and organizing interdisciplinary knowledge. In *Health Through Occupation*, G Kielhofner, Editor. Philadelphia: FA Davis Company, 1983
8. Kielhofner G, Burke JP: Components and determinants of human occupation. In *A Model of Human Occupation*, G. Kielhofner, Editor, Baltimore: Williams & Wilkins, 1985
9. Hamilton C: The effectiveness of an occupational therapy program in the develop-

ment of maternal competence in primiparous mothers of fullterm infants. Unpublished masters thesis. University of Southern California, 1983

10. Kawamoto T: Satisfaction with a maternal preparation program received in conjunction with obstetric care. Unpublished masters thesis, USC, 1983

11. Smart M, Smart R: *Infants, Development and Relationships* . New York: MacMillan, 1973

12. Day S: Mother-infant activities as sensory stimulation. *Am J Occup Ther* 36:579-585, 1982

13. Ayres AJ: *Sensory Integration and the child.* Los Angeles: Western Psychological Services, 1983

14. Heard C: Occupational role acquisition: a perspective on the chronically disabled. *Am J Occup Ther* 31:243-247, 1977

15. Sandberg ED: *Synopsis of Obstetrics* [10th edition] St. Louis: CV Mosby Co. 1978

Evaluation of Praxis
in Preschoolers

L. Diane Parham, MA, OTR

SUMMARY. This article draws from the research and clinical work of A. Jean Ayres to present a rationale and set of procedures for occupational therapy evaluation of the preschooler whose presenting problems suggest dyspraxia. The concept of praxis is briefly discussed and the problems of evaluating praxis in the preschooler are outlined. Based on the literature in this area, two major domains for evaluation are examined: sensory processing and praxis. In the domain of sensory processing, special attention is given to assessment of tactile, proprioceptive, vestibular, auditory, and visual functions. The domain of praxis is organized according to three primary processes: ideation, motor planning, and execution. Procedures for each domain are suggested, including administration of standardized test items, parent interviews, and structured observations, as well as observation of behavior in unstructured situations. Precautions in interpretation of data and suggestions for presenting evaluation findings in the clinical report are delineated. Finally, consideration is given to issues related to recommendation of occupational therapy, referral to other professionals, and setting of treatment goals for the dyspraxic child.

Occupational therapists working with preschoolers are centrally concerned with the child's ability to organize and participate in play and self-care activities. According to the sensory integrative per-

L. Diane Parham is Director of Education, The Ayres Clinic, Torrance, California and Assistant Professor, Occupational Therapy, University of Southern California, Los Angeles, CA.

This paper is based on a briefer article by the author entitled "Assessment: The Preschooler with Suspected Dyspraxia," published by the American Occupational Therapy Association in the *Sensory Integration Special Interest Section Newsletter*, Volume 9, Number 1, March, 1986.

This article appears jointly in *Sensory Integrative Approaches in Occupational Therapy* (The Haworth Press, 1987) and *Occupational Therapy in Health Care*, Volume 4, Number 2 (Summer 1987).

23

spective of Ayres, such activities place a demand on praxis, an underlying ability that is basic to human transactions with the physical environment.[1] Because practicability is developing rapidly in the early years of life, and because it critically influences the child's performance in daily activities, the evaluation of praxis is an important element of occupational therapy practice with preschoolers.

Referrals for occupational therapy evaluation of preschoolers may indicate presenting problems suggestive of poorly developed praxis. Examples of such problems include: "unable to organize playing by himself," "doesn't know what to do with toys and often breaks them," "wants to join other children on the playground but can't do the activities unless given a lot of help from adults," "loves to ride her rocking horse but repeatedly has to be helped step by step to get on, and then cannot figure out how to get off," or "has a lot of difficulty putting on clothes and is now beginning to have tantrums habitually when asked to do so." In many cases a language delay is present. Some of these children are overly active and oblivious to danger, but others seem unusually fearful and reluctant to become involved in ordinary gross motor play activities. When presenting problems such as these occur in a child whose intelligence is within normal limits and whose daily environment provides a variety of stimulating opportunities for development of motor ability, the possibility of dyspraxia should be considered by the therapist. Evaluation procedures, then, can be designed to investigate this possibility.

Although developmental dyspraxia classically occurs in children who do not have neuromotor disabilities, it can coexist with a neuromotor diagnosis, such as cerebral palsy. The therapist must be sensitive to the fact that some individuals with cerebral palsy have a well developed practicability. Consider the following portrait of Paul, an adult who uses praxis exquisitely to compensate for severe athetosis. Although Kielhofner[2] does not identify Paul's ability as praxis, his description provides us with a vivid case example:

> It is amazing to watch Paul eat. I have the feeling that if I were given his body at this moment, I would be absolutely unable to do anything useful with it. Despite all its writhings and distortions, Paul's body does all the things it has to and the care with which he organizes and executes each movement is striking. Paul is a truly graceful cerebral palsied person. It is near mystery to watch him wind his unruly hands around a cup of tea

which is purposefully not too hot so as not to burn him should a sudden involuntary movement dump it into his mouth or over his face. He slowly places one hand toward the cup, nudging it with the other to focus the movement. When his hand is in place, he makes a grasping movement which sends off a whole parade of involuntary contractions throughout his arm. The second hand is still steadying things during all this. Then, the second hand moves just as carefully to embrace the other one. Now, with this two-handed grasp in which his fingers literally encircle and hide the cup, he brings his face and hands to meet halfway and sips the tea with lips and throat that move uncontrollably. The tea spills, he makes gurgling loud sipping noises and chokes a bit on the tea. In the midst of all this, Paul remains impeccably calm and dignified. [2,p.83-84]

In some cerebral palsied individuals, however, purposeful activity is hindered to an extent beyond what can be explained by the neuromotor disability alone, possibly due to the concomitant presence of dyspraxia. While a neuromotor problem interferes with precise execution of specific motor acts, dyspraxia interferes with the organization of functional behavior in a broader sense. It impedes the person's conceptualization of how to organize actions effectively.

THE PROBLEM: HOW TO EVALUATE, HOW TO INTERPRET

Evaluation of praxis in children is a relatively new area with little clinical literature published to date. The advent of the soon to be published Sensory Integration and Praxis Test (SIPT) [3] will be a boon to the clinician interested in this area. In the meantime, evaluation is difficult and the clinician must rely to a great extent on clinical observation. It is particularly difficult if the patient is a young preschooler for whom there are few age-appropriate tests. In the case of the SIPT, normative data will be available only for preschoolers who are at least four years of age. Even when other standardized tests are available, preschoolers are notoriously difficult to test, and test scores for this age group tend to be weak in reliability. To skillfully assess these youngsters, the therapist must develop sharp observational skills and draw interpretations from knowledge of existing theory and research on the nature of praxis and developmental dyspraxia.

In this article, some suggestions will be made regarding how a therapist might structure an evaluation of a preschooler with presenting signs of dyspraxia, and how evaluation results might be interpreted. Suggestions presented here are guided by the recent works of Ayres[1] on developmental dyspraxia. The reader is referred to this source for theoretical and research background. To briefly summarize research in this area, developmental dyspraxia has been found to be closely related to poor somatosensory processing, particularly tactile perception. Development of praxis appears to be intimately tied to perceptual and language development.[1,4-9] Although different facets of praxis can be identified (constructional, oral, postural, etc.), Ayres believes that praxis is essentially a unitary function that involves three basic processes: *ideation*, or generating an idea of how one might interact with the environment, *motor planning*, or organizing a program of action, and *execution*, the actual performance of a motor act.[1] Ayres hypothesizes that somatosensory processing is a critical function in the development of praxis, particularly with respect to the ideation or concept formation component.[1]

SUGGESTED EVALUATION PROCEDURES

The literature outlined above suggests that evaluation should address two primary domains: sensory processing and praxis. Within each domain, specific areas of functioning should be evaluated (discussed below). When the SIPT is available, it will be ideally suited for detailed evaluation of these domains in testable four to five year olds. For many preschoolers, however, testing with the SIPT will be inappropriate or unfeasible and the clinician will have to rely on skilled observation. Observing the child in a clinical setting with therapeutic equipment which affords a variety of sensory and motor experiences is recommended. Spontaneous play should be observed as well as reactions to structured situations. A parent interview often provides key information regarding past development and present functional problems.

When appropriate and feasible, standardized tests can be administered. It can be advantageous to select certain items from published tests, particularly if the child is unable or unwilling to cooperate with more extensive testing. This is most helpful when normative data, such as percentile scores, for the child's age level are provided on individual items or subtests. Reliability of obtained scores must always be considered. Of course, single item scores provide very circumscribed information and are usually limited in reliability. Nevertheless, judicious use of individual test items or subtest scores, together with other supporting data, can be helpful in clarifying the nature of the problem in a young child who is otherwise untestable.

Specific procedures that can be used are suggested in the following sections. Most are derived from the work of Ayres. They are grouped according to the two primary domains of interest, sensory processing and praxis.

Sensory Processing

A sensory history provided by the parent can furnish clues regarding auditory, visual, olfactory, gustatory, vestibular, and somatosensory functions. More in-depth examination, particularly of somatosensory and vestibular processing, is recommended in the clinical setting.

Tactile Processing. In the realm of tactile perception and modulation, consider the following: Does the child seem to seek out or avoid certain tactile experiences? Are behaviors suggestive of tactile defensiveness observed? Can the child find a small toy hidden in a "feely box" (for example, a box filled with styrofoam packing material, rice, plastic bubble balls, or dried beans)? When a puff of air is applied to the back of the child's neck unexpectedly, does the child orient to the stimulus? Does the child orient to other light tactile stimuli (such as from cotton puff or pencil eraser) applied unexpectedly and out of visual field? If the child falls or suffers a minor physical injury, is there any evidence of pain reaction? Does the child overreact to minor bumps and falls? Interview the caregiver and probe for information related to reactions to touch and pain sensations.

Administration of the Stereognosis and Finger Localization items from the Miller Assessment for Preschoolers (MAP)[10] may provide useful data. The stereognosis test developed by Tyler[11] is an alternative. When administering stereognosis tests, watch to see if the child initiates active, exploratory touch strategies. Even if a score is not obtained, an important observation is whether or not the child spontaneously manipulates test objects purposefully to obtain tactile information when visual cues are absent. Fine dexterity in general can provide an indicator of whether or not tactile sensations are being used optimally to guide movement.

Proprioceptive Processing. This is more difficult to evaluate because of the confounding effects of vestibular and neuromotor functions, which must be weighed when interpreting observations. Balance, postural reactions, postural background movements, cocontraction, and quality of total body patterns (flexion, extension, rotation) can provide clues to functioning in this area. Does the child habitually assume body positions that place joints in extreme ends of range of motion (for example, sitting or standing with hips in extreme internal rotation)? When the child rides on a piece of equipment, such as scooter board or bolster swing, is there automatic positioning of the trunk for optimal stability? What is the quality of postural adjustments when they are made? Is it easy to manually facilitate the child to change body position, or is there a relative lack of responsiveness? When moving to sit on a surface, step over an object, or stoop under an obstacle, does the child seem unsure of how far to raise or lower body parts? Administration of the Postural Control subtest of the DeGangi-Berk Test of Sensory Integration (TSI)[12] may provide a useful means of systematically documenting performance on tasks that are related to proprioceptive functioning, such as neck and arm cocontraction. Vertical Writing and Hand-Nose from the MAP can provide additional information. Keep in mind that performance on these kinds of tasks can be heavily influenced by unusual or abnormal patterns of muscle tone that may be reflective of neuromotor disorder rather than poor proprioception per se.

Vestibular Processing. The influence of vestibular processing must be considered when assessing the proprioceptive tasks mentioned above. More direct measures of vestibular functions can also be included, for example, observation or testing of postrotary nystagmus. In many research studies the duration of this normal vestibulo-ocular reflex has discriminated between children with developmental problems and those with normal development.[13] Thus, it provides a gross index of developmental status with regard to visual-vestibular sensory integrative functions.

Research by Deitz, Siegner, and Crowe[14] indicated that the Southern California Postrotary Nystagmus Test[15] can be administered reliably to four-year olds. The means and standard deviations from their study can be used as a guide for interpretation of this test with this age group. However, their data on three-year-olds indicated that this test is not reliable enough for administration to these younger children. Even so, it can be appropriate to observe for the presence of perrotary and postrotary nystagmus in younger children. Perrotary nystagmus refers to observable nystagmus during body rotation, while postrotary nystagmus refers to observable nystagmus after cessation of body rotation. Review of research indicates that perrotary and postrotary nystagmus are easily observed in normally developing infants beyond four to five months of age when rotation has been given for longer than 10 seconds. [11] Thus, even if a score is not obtainable, noting the presence of these normal oculoreflexive responses provides a gross indicator of vestibular functioning. Rotation can be given gently and playfully while the child is sitting supported in a platform swing or other piece of suspended equipment. Absence of any observable nystagmic responses to rotation is very unusual and could be a sign of delayed or abnormal maturation of vestibular functioning.

Other indicators of vestibular processing that could be observed include quality of equilibrium responses, righting reactions, protective arm extension, prone extension during linear acceleration, and postural reactions when moving against gravity (for example, walking up an incline). Relevant MAP items are the Romberg, Stepping, and Walks Line. As bilateral coordination has been theoretically linked with vestibular processing, the therapist may wish to include observations or tests of bilateral coordination, such as the Bilateral Motor Coordination subtest of the TSI and the Rapid Alternating Movements (Stamp) item of the MAP. Eye pursuits can be observed as well. The therapist should keep in mind that most of these observations do not solely reflect function of the vestibular system.

Affective responses to vestibular input should be noted. Clinical experience indicates that most normal preschoolers, by about three years of age, react with obvious delight to the vestibular sensations afforded by suspended equipment and climbing apparatuses. When a child reacts to gentle movement through space with an unusual degree of overt anxiety or fear, the possibility of gravitational insecurity should be considered. How does the child react when tipped backward? This can be done with the child supine over a bolster or simply held in the arms of the examiner. Gravitationally insecure children react aversively to this sensation, e.g., they may cry, startle, cling tightly to the adult, and otherwise appear very uncomfortable or disturbed. Usually these children avoid climbing and other gross motor activities that require them to lift their feet away from the floor in a manner that is different from habitual walking. They also tend to avoid unstable surfaces, such as mats or tiltboards, and seem insecure when moving from one surface to another, as when stepping from mats to linoleum floor. Vertical linear sensations, in particular, seem discomforting, and often the child will avoid moving the head in a plane that is different from the usual upright position. When fearful reactions are manifested, the therapist should attempt to discover whether a true gravitational insecurity is present, i.e., negative response to gravity sensations. Sometimes a child who enjoys being moved in different planes at different intensities will appear apprehensive or fearful when faced with a motor task that demands active planning. It may be that the fear is a result of having learned to anticipate failure. Rather than demonstrating grativational insecurity such a child may lack confidence.

Visual and Auditory Processing. The therapist should observe the types of visual and auditory stimuli to which the child orients. Does he or she attend to the sight of moving objects or children, or to novel equipment in the room? Do visual exploration and searching occur? Simple items from the MAP (Puzzle, Figure-Ground) may aid in assessing visual perception. Is the child responsive to speech sounds? Is there an alerting reaction to any unusual sounds that may occur? Does the child seem generally oblivious to the surrounding visual or auditory stimuli? Barring any deficit in visual or hearing acuity, this could suggest a problem in sensory registration, which involves selectively orienting and paying attention to environmental stimuli in an adaptive manner. At the opposite extreme is a sensory registration problem in which too much orienting occurs — the child attends to one stimulus after another, resulting in constant movement, distractibility, and difficulty sustaining attention on a single task.

Praxis

The three processes of ideation, motor planning, and execution (defined earlier in this paper) should be addressed during evaluation. Observation of motor activity is basic to evaluating all three processes.

Ideation. Ideation can be difficult to assess. Since no objective tests exist to tap this construct, it is highly inferential. One of the best ways to evaluate this ability is to observe the way the child plays spontaneously with toys and therapeutic equipment. It is particularly revealing to observe what is done with novel equipment that has never been seen before by the child. Initially, do not direct the child. The goal here is to gain insight into the extent to which the child can generate and organize ideas of what to do.

Does the child anticipate the potential for riding, swinging, or climbing in a variety of ways on equipment designed for whole body action? If very active, is the child goal-directed and purposeful? Randomly pushing separate pieces of equipment around the room, without any constructive relating of one piece to another, may indicate difficulty with ideation. Some children with poor ideation resort to throwing objects or toys, at times aggressively. Often, three- to four-year old dyspraxic children with poor ideation will do a simple action repeatedly without elaboration, for example, running up and down a ramp. Others will not initiate any action with equipment unless explicitly directed. When this occurs, the therapist should attempt to sort out whether this is due primarily to poor ideation or under-registration of sensory information. Children who fail to register much of the sensory world around them will usually have poor ideation, but poor ideation does not necessarily imply poor registration. When dealing with a culturally different child, the possibility must also be considered that the child may have been taught to await direction or permission before actively playing in an unfamiliar situation or in the presence of an unfamiliar adult.

Motor Planning. Sometimes a child will seem to have an idea of what can be done, and may even be able to verbally express the desired action, but cannot organize body parts to effectively execute the action. The child may have a problem in motor planning. An example is a three-year old girl who wanted to ride on a scooter board. Instead of going through the sequence of motions that would bring her into a prone position on the board, she simply stood next to it, stepping in place repeatedly. Because she was unable to generate an adequate motor plan, she had resorted to using centrally programmed movements which were inappropriate for the task. Eventually she had to be physically guided to lie on the scooter board.

It may be difficult to distinguish a specific problem in motor planning from an ideation problem. Usually, a child with poor ideation will have poor motor planning, since the nature of the task at hand is not grasped. The picture may be clarified by providing the child with cues of how to do the task, such as watching another child doing the activity. If the problem is primarily limited to ideation, the child will be able to imitate adequately. It is more common to find that the child with poor ideation generally has difficulty organizing actions even when provided with verbal and demonstrated instructions. Moreover, this kind of child may not readily generalize a motor plan from one situation to another. That is, the child may be able to motor plan a specific task in one situation, but when presented with a similar task in a different situation, is not able to organize a response adequately.

To supplement observations, testing can sometimes be conducted to provide further information on motor planning. Therapists trained in the SIPT may choose to administer parts of the praxis tests as an informal method for evaluating motor planning in preschoolers who are younger than the standardization sample. Of course, numerical scores cannot be obtained or interpreted with confidence when this is done. Some MAP items also may be helpful in this area: Block Tapping (sequencing praxis), Block Designs (constructional praxis), Draw-A-Person (graphic praxis), Imitate Postures (postural praxis), Tongue Movements (oral praxis), and Maze (manual praxis).

Execution. Ayres[1] points out that when problems of motor execution are observed, the therapist should analyze the possibility that the difficulties could be due to either poor ideation or limited motor planning. Motor execution can also be impeded by a neuromotor involvement, such as abnormal patterns of muscle tone, tremor, choreoform movements, obligatory primitive reflexes, or motor impersistence. The impact of these, if present, should be assessed. More detailed evaluation of neuromotor problems can be initiated if deemed necessary.

PRESENTING EVALUATION RESULTS

The clinical report will usually be written in narrative form. Since evaluation of dyspraxic preschoolers relies so heavily on clinical judgment, results must be presented cautiously. It is mandatory that the therapist be well grounded in relevant theory and research. The work of Ayres[1] and Cermak[16] on dyspraxia, as well as the views of experts from other professions[17-19] should be familiar to the occupational therapist who evaluates praxis in children. It is recommended that the guidelines for interpretation of praxis performance suggested by Ayres[1] be reviewed carefully. Before the SIPT is used, the therapist should complete the education process leading to certification by Sensory Integration International in the administration and interpretation of these tests.

If a test is used that yields a score of questionable reliability, as is often the case with preschoolers, it is probably best to interpret performance in qualitative terms. In such cases, the therapist should use normative data as a general guide rather than putting emphasis on specific numerical scores. Performance on tests should also be integrated with observational and historical data. For example, one might write something like the following:

> John was unable to score any points on the Tongue Movements item of the MAP, a poor performance for a child his age. This finding, together with the history of eating problems and the reported inability to adequately chew foods with uneven texture, suggests that oral praxis may be an area of particular difficulty for him.

Constructs such as praxis should be defined for the reader in the report prior to discussion. Giving concrete examples of what was observed can also be enlightening for the reader. Here is an example:

> Praxis refers to the ability to form an idea about an action, plan the action, and execute the motions necessary to carry out the action. This was assessed by observing Bonnie's approach to a variety of unfamiliar activities. Bonnie readily approached novel therapeutic equipment and seemed eager to engage in play, thereby showing some degree of ideation. However, she seemed to have considerable difficulty with the motor planning aspect of praxis. She tended to spontaneously use habitual patterns of walking, standing, or sitting with very little variation when interacting with equipment. Bonnie was generally accepting of the therapist's directions to try new positions or activities, but she required extensive physical assistance. For example, she needed step-by-step physical assistance in order to get on and off a suspended platform swing. She was unable to propel a scooterboard with hands while prone despite physical guidance and repeated attempts. On MAP

items, she performed well on Imitation of Postures, which requires imitation of simple arm positions, but she was unable to imitate a half-kneel position for Kneel-Stand until given physical guidance. It appeared that the trunk rotation involved in this body position, as well as the motor planning required to assume it, gave her considerable difficulty.

The evaluating therapist should make recommendations regarding whether or not occupational therapy is appropriate, and if it is, which types of treatment procedures should be used. When there is evidence of dyspraxia along with neuromotor or orthopedic problems, occupational therapy might be recommended using sensory integrative procedures, neurodevelopmental techniques, provision of adaptive equipment, and/or training in compensatory strategies. In the case of the child who demonstrates clear evidence of dyspraxia or other sensory integrative problems without neuromotor involvement, occupational therapy using sensory integrative procedures may be the treatment of choice. This is particularly important for the severely dyspraxic child, as severe dyspraxia does not seem to improve over time without intervention.[20] Moreover, children with mild dyspraxia continue to have difficulty with some motor tasks if no intervention is given, although natural improvement may take place to some extent.[20] The presence of concomitant behavior or language problems would also implicate the importance of early initiation of therapy. Most experts in the field of developmental dyspraxia recommend occupational therapy as a valuable and appropriate treatment.[17,18] Gubbay specifically recommends sensory integrative procedures, and states that prognosis is excellent if a dyspraxic child with good intelligence is given therapy at an early age.[18]

A referral for evaluation by other professionals should be recommended if relevant. For example, referral to a physician for consideration of medication might be made if hyperactivity or lack of sustained attention is a significant problem. For selected cases, referrals to speech pathologists, physical therapists, and other occupational therapists with expertise in specific problem areas could be considered.

When occupational therapy is recommended, the report usually designates general goals of treatment as well as appropriate procedures. If sensory integrative procedures are used for a dyspraxic child, goals will probably be directed toward improving ideation and/or motor planning ability, depending on the characteristics of the child. Goals may also relate to particular sensory processing difficulties if indicated by evaluation results. Ultimately, therapy is aimed at making a positive impact on the child's occupational performance, so long range goals should anticipate changes in areas such as behavioral organization at home and in preschool, self-care and communication skills, self-confidence, social skills, and ability to participate in developmentally more complex play activities. Interviewing the caregivers regarding initial problems seen in these areas, and conducting more extensive evaluation of those that appear most compromised, can aid the therapist in targeting behaviors that may change over the course of intervention. If therapy is initiated, it will be most important to plan and instate a system for measuring change from the very beginning. Although direct measures of praxis ability can be used, it will be the more functional, broader aspects of occupational performance that will reflect whether or not therapy has truly made an impact on the individual child's quality of life.

REFERENCES

1. Ayres, AJ: *Developmental Dyspraxia and Adult Onset Apraxia*. Torrance, CA, Sensory Integration International, 1985

2. Kielhofner, G: *Health Through Occupation – Theory and Practice in Occupational Therapy*. Philadelphia, FA Davis, 1983

3. Ayres, AJ: *Sensory Integration and Praxis Tests*. Los Angeles, Western Psychological Services, in preparation

4. Ayres, AJ: Patterns of perceptual-motor dysfunction in children: A factor analytic study. *Perceptual and Motor Skills* 20: 335-368, 1965

5. Ayres, AJ: Interrelationships among perceptual-motor functions in children. *Amer J Occup Ther* 20: 68-71, 1966

6. Ayres, AJ: Deficits in sensory integration in educationally handicapped children. *J Learning Dis* 2: 160-168, 1969

7. Ayres, AJ: Cluster analyses of measures of sensory integration. *Am J Occup Ther* 31: 362-366, 1977

8. Ayres, AJ, Mailloux, ZK, & Wendler, CLW: Developmental dyspraxia: Is it a unitary function? Paper presented at Sensory Integration Symposium, sponsored by Sensory Integration International, Boston, 1985

9. Gubbay, SS, Ellis, E, Walton, JN, & Court, SDM: Clumsy children: A study of apraxic and agnostic defects in 21 children. *Brain* 88: 295-312, 1965

10. Miller, LJ: *Miller Assessment for Preschoolers*. Littleton, CO, Foundation for Knowledge in Development, 1982

11. Tyler, N: A stereognostic test for screening tactile sensation. *Am J Occup Ther* 26: 256-260, 1972

12. Berk, RA & DeGangi, GA: *DeGangi-Berk Test of Sensory Integration*. Los Angeles, Western Psychological Services, 1983

13. Ornitz, EM: Normal and pathological maturation of vestibular function in the human child, in Romand, R. (ed): *Development of Auditory and Vestibular Systems*, New York, Academic, pp. 479-536, 1983

14. Deitz, JC, Siegner, CB, & Crowe, TK: The Southern California Postrotary Nystagmus Test: Test-retest reliability for preschool children. *Occup Ther J Research* 1: 165-177, 1981

15. Ayres, AJ: *Southern California Postrotary Nystagmus Test*. Los Angeles, Western Psychological Services, 1981

16. Cermak, S: Developmental dyspraxia, in Roy, EA (ed): *Neuropsychological Studies of Apraxia and Related Disorders*, Amsterdam, Netherlands, Elsevier, pp. 225-248, 1985

17. Dawdy, SC: Pediatric neuropsychology: Caring for the developmentally dyspraxic child. *Clinical Neuropsychology* 3: 30-37, 1981

18. Gubbay, SS: The management of developmental apraxia. *Dev Med Child Neuro* 20: 643-646, 1978

19. Roy, EA (ed): *Neuropsychological Studies of Apraxia and Related Disorders*. Amsterdam, Netherlands, Elsevier, 1985

20. Knuckey, NW & Gubbay, SS: Clumsy children: A prognostic study. *Aust Pediatr J* 19: 9-13, 1983

Movement Is Fun:
An Occupational Therapy Perspective
on a Program for Preschoolers

Susan B. Young, MA, OTR, FAOTA

SUMMARY. A movement program for children based on sensory integration theory, using movement education concepts, was developed by an occupational therapist for use in preschool settings. The goal of the program is to enhance normal growth and development in 3-5 year old children, and to provide a vehicle for early identification of children with developmental delays. The paper will describe the curriculum and provide examples of activities used as well as suggestions for instituting such a program elsewhere. Research has not been conducted on the effects of the program, but comments from teachers, parents and therapists involved indicate that the program is meeting its goals.

Sensory integrative function and development is a normal process which occurs in every developing child. Occupational therapists have tended to focus on sensory integrative *dys*function when utilizing the sensory integrative framework in clinics. Treatment programs enhance and normalize the processing of sensory information so that an appropriate adaptive response can be made. If there is an interruption in the development of sensory integrative function, it appears to be best to identify it early and begin remediation immediately.

Susan B. Young is Director and a practicing therapist in a private practice, Children's Therapy Group, Leawood, KS.

Acknowledgement: The author wishes to thank Liz Keplinger for her devotion and contributions to the development of this program.

This article appears jointly in *Sensory Integrative Approaches in Occupational Therapy* (The Haworth Press, 1987) and *Occupational Therapy in Health Care*, Volume 4, Number 2 (Summer 1987).

37

Movement Is Fun (MIF) is a program developed by an occupational therapist to enhance sensory processing abilities in preschoolers. Since occupational therapists have education in neurobiology as well as activity analysis and selection, they seem to be in a unique position to design a program of activities to enhance sensory processing. In addition, sensory integration theory has become an important part of the evaluation and remediation repertoire of many occupational therapists. Thus, this curriculum uses sensory integration theory as a framework on which fun activities have been designed.

Early identification of children who may be having motor or sensory processing problems is easily accomplished as the therapist conducts the sessions and observes the children in once a week sessions. Using the observational skills needed to evaluate children in the clinic to recognize movement problems, defensive responses to the sensory input and changes in arousal level caused by the activities, the therapist can identify problems needing further evaluation. The added benefit of being in the school and a part of the staff creates visibility for the therapist and facilitates interaction which seems to lead to utilization of sensory integration concepts in the classroom. Therapist accessibility also allows for questions and answers concerning specific children in the school.

HISTORY AND PURPOSE

Since its early years, a large church affiliated preschool in Kansas City has incorporated motor development objectives as part of its curriculum. The curriculum recognized the importance of movement and motor development as a basis for children acquiring higher conceptual skills. For example, prepositional phrases (behind, above, below, etc.) were incorporated in the class "motor development time" through using music, following the directions given on commercially available records. Concepts being covered in the classroom curriculum, such as geometric shapes, were encouraged in movement sessions as was directing the children to explore space through movement.

The author was associated with the school and had been involved in consulting with the school for several years when the school's director decided to increase the motor development aspect of the curriculum. She suggested at that time that the therapist be responsible, in conjunction with the preschool staff, for developing and carrying out a movement curriculum which would be incorporated into the total school program and which eventually classroom teachers could carry out with consultation by the therapist.

The sensory integration development theory hypothesized by A. Jean Ayres[1] was chosen as the framework for the program for the following reasons:

1. The concept of enhancing normal growth and development through concepts utilized in treating dysfunctioning children seemed both intriguing and appropriate.
2. Sensory integration techniques are for the most part carried out on an individual basis. However, many therapists see small groups in treatment; there seemed to be a need to develop activities which could be used therapeutically with small groups. (MIF was not designed to be used as therapy or as a substitute for individual therapy but some of the activities may be incorporated into therapeutic programs.)
3. The components of this theory are very sequential and theoretically culminate in the acquisition of academic skills.
4. Employing sensory motor activities in a group situation would tend to help the therapist identify children whose sensory processing systems were immature or dysfunctioning. At this age level, that could mean early discovery of problems.

The curriculum was written in an educational format, i.e., lesson plans, that classroom teachers might be able to learn and use the program in their schools, preferably with occupational therapy consultation.

One of the professionals working with the school described above was a teacher of adaptive physical education interested in developing movement activities for young children. Her approach utilized movement exploration concepts. Many of her ideas were invaluable in setting up the activities and approaches within a sensory integration based program. Her skill at working with groups of children and knowing how to manage the class merged well with the therapist's knowledge of sensory integration theory and neurobiology to provide a program which met the objectives of both the school and the author.

GENERAL THEORY AND STRUCTURE

The MIF program has sought to mesh elements of movement education programs with the theory of sensory integration development. Since the goal of the program is to enhance normal growth and development, normal developmental stages have been followed and integrated into the structure of the curriculum.

Movement education literature seems to be written by and for physical educators. Goals and objectives of such programs include teaching the use of the body in space, stimulating the spirit of exploration in space, problem solving body movement, body awareness, timing of movements, weight and force of movement, flow of movement.[2,3] Most programs include working on specific skills such as balancing, skipping, balance beam, jumping and the use of the ball. Occasionally music is used. These programs encourage and allow the child to concentrate on his body as it moves and to learn about his body and how it relates to the environment around him. Creativity and problem solving is stimulated by the teacher using such words as "show me how . . . ," "can you find another way . . . ," "how many different ways can you . . . ," when directing the children's activity.[3] Movement education or movement exploration programs are often directed by a physical education teacher and are generally used with preschool and elementary age children.

Ayres has hypothesized that development of basic sensory systems and the integration of information in the brain is necessary before higher level skills will appear and be normal.[4] She has identified the main sensory systems as vestibular (information about gravity and space), proprioceptive (information about muscles and joints) and tactile (information about things in the environment that touch you). If these three systems are working well, then motor development and higher level functions such as academic skills will automatically build on this base and develop normally.

It is this developmental aspect of the theory of sensory integrations that was used as the basis of this curriculum. Superimposed on this framework are many of the concepts inherent in movement education programs.

The MIF program is conducted in the school, by the therapists and teachers who are trained by the therapist, for children ages 3-5. Each class (11-18 children with shoes and socks removed) is brought to "the movement room" by one of their teachers. The movement room is carpeted, large enough for all the children to move freely and has no obstacles. Because of the change of focus in the movement activities from that expected in the classroom, a different room seems to make it easier for the children to move freely. There have been instances when the activities were conducted in the classroom but this was not as successful. One classroom teacher and the movement leader participate in the activities. Each class participates once a week for 30 minutes throughout the school year. Equipment is kept to a minimum so that the focus of the child will be on his body and space rather than on equipment. A record player, records, hula hoops, balloons, balls, mats, and beanbags are examples of equipment used.

There are few rules in conducting the session, but those that exist are primarily for safety. They include:

1. When the MIF teacher claps twice, everyone "freezes like a statue."
2. When moving around the room, no one touches his neighbor or the room walls unless directed to do so.
3. Only one person can talk at a time and the MIF leader takes precedence.
4. All people in the room participate, including adults, so that no person becomes an obstacle. (This also encourages freer participation by the children.)

Close management of the class is very important with so many young children moving around. For maximum control, directions are generally given with the children seated. Young children seem to have difficulty listening when they are standing. Positive reinforcement for moving, especially doing creative movement within the activity objective is lavishly given. General commands are avoided such as "Go line up" because that tends to cause running. Instead, the MIF leader might say, "When I touch you on the head, you may line up."

Each class period is divided into three sections, i.e., warm-up, activities which meet the day's objective and cool-down. The warm-up activities are usually done to music and involve moving around the room in various ways. The day's objectives are met by designing activities which all the children can do and which stimulate specific sensory processing. The cool-down time involves the children in relaxation prior to going back to the classroom. They are taught about warming-up before exercise as a healthy habit and of letting one's body cool-down after exercise. They are always encouraged to explore the various ways their bodies move and praised for thinking of a different way rather than the sameness that is often reinforced in regular classrooms.

UNITS AND EXAMPLES

The six units in the curriculum follow the developmental continuum which Ayres has used in describing the sensory-motor development process.[4] Unit objectives and examples of activities are as follows:

1. *Tactile* — These activities include those for general stimulation in conjunction with movement, as well as discrimination tasks. For example, the children are asked to move like a worm on the carpet to music (Walter the Waltzing Worm[5]). Another activity involves pulling "tubes" of cloth on their bodies and wiggling out of the tube on their tummies, or on their backs, or going up or going down while a partner helps hold the tube. Another example is to suggest a "pretend trip" to the ocean. Children "swim" on the carpet, then dry off different body parts with their "towel" which is carpet. They are directed as to which body parts they need to put on the carpeted floor and then to rub it dry. A discrimination task involves the children sitting in a children's pool filled with styrofoam packing and matching and identifying objects while wearing a mask. Such objects as blocks, pegs, or shapes are used.

2. *Vestibular* — Movement involving spinning, rolling and shaking of the head are included. One example is to have the children pretending to be tops spinning on the floor. Different positions in which to spin are encouraged (stomach, back, hips). This is done to music called "Spinning, Spinning Like a Top."[6] Another example is to suggest children pretend to be a rocking horse and rock in different positions to music. Rolling activities include pretending to be logs rolling up and down a mountain made of mats, or being a bowling ball and knocking over pins (cardboard blocks), or being an Easter egg and rolling around the "yard." The song, "Shake Something," from the "Getting To Know Myself" record[6] is used for shaking of the head to stimulate vestibular receptors.

3. *Proprioceptive* — Heavy work activities are used. An example is having each child pull on a rubber stretchie (1" wide loops of rubber cut from inner tubes) with different body parts. Directions

are given such as "Pull the stretchie with one hand and one knee" or "Pull on the stretchie above your head with two hands." Tug-of-war is a heavy work activity and is also used. Another time, the children pretend to "ice skate" on the carpet to music with the stretchie around their ankles. In one lesson, the children take a "sleigh ride" on a folded up mat with a rope attached. Other children are "horses" and pull the sleigh. The children also pretend to be turtles and move around with beanbag chairs on their backs.

4. *Postural* — Activities for trunk extension, trunk flexion and static and dynamic balance are included. An example is having a child do "egg rolls" down a mat for flexion or lying on their backs and rocking backward and forward while holding on to their knees. For extension, they may lie on their stomachs and roll a ball to a partner across from them or pass balls backwards over their heads to a child behind. Balance activities include balancing on different body parts, i.e., one foot, balancing a beanbag on different body parts and walking, knee walking and crawling on "a masking tape road" (strips of tape on the carpet). Some obstacle courses which have balance beams in them are also used.

5. *Bilateral* — Movement which involves using both sides of the body simultaneously are included in this section of the program. An example is using a parachute in different ways such as raising and lowering it with both hands on the handles, or doing hopscotch on carpet squares using jumps with feet apart and then feet together instead of hops. Balloons are used in one lesson with the children hitting them up into the air with two hands, playing catch with a friend or bouncing them on the floor and catching them.

6. *Motor skill development* — Ball and jump rope skills are begun as well as some aerobic dancing (following directions given to music). In addition, getting children to follow commands of a much more complex nature is included. An example is having them bounce, throw and catch a ball. Teaching jump rope is begun first by introducing jump rope rhythm using a confined area such as a carpet square to jump on ("jump *and* jump *and* jump"). Children then jump rope with teachers turning the rope. Finally they progress to using a hula hoop as "a jump rope" which they "turn" by themselves. Movement music is used, such as the record, "Pre-Square Dance"[8] which involves doing a circle dance following the voice on the record.

Warm-up activities done to music consist of free movement time with the MIF leader giving general directions such as "move backwards," "move sideways." *Cool-down* activities involve slow, quiet things such as "pretend to be a snowflake gently floating to the ground" followed by lying quietly until touched by the teacher to line up for return to the classroom. Quiet music helps the children to relax.

Throughout the curriculum, motor planning is required along with auditory-motor responses. While the leaders are a part of the group, they do not demonstrate the activities; they ask the children to so that the children must make their own plan instead of imitating. For example, if the concept is making the body be like a top that is spinning, the MIF leader might ask, "How can you make your body spin like a top?" Once a child demonstrates a method, she then asks, "How else can you make your body spin like a top?" This requires that the child plan and carry out a new motor task without seeing it demonstrated. Another example would be the instruction "Balance on two hands and one knee." "Balance on your head and two feet." The children hear the direction, picture it in their minds and then carry out the task which is then regarded by positive reinforcement from the leader.

EVALUATION

The initial hypothesis for the MIF program was that normal growth and development would be enhanced by designing a movement program based on sensory integration theory. Although a research project was designed to test this, it was not completed in part because both the school and the parents were unwilling to have a control group that excluded some children from participation. However, it is believed that a research protocol could be designed which might begin to assess the benefit of this kind of curriculum.

Anecdotal data from the experience include frequent parent and teacher comments which have been used as informal assessments of the program. Teachers report that person drawings are consistently more mature about 4-5 months after the child is in the program. Since at the pilot school neither curriculum nor teachers had changed significantly since the program began, results appear to be attributed to the activities. Teachers also report children show improved orientation to space, such as in lining up, moving through the classroom and in following directions by placing forms on a paper during craft time. Parents report that their children carry over many of the activities at home, dance and move freely to music, often saying that it is "like in movement class." Both parents and teachers report that the children frequently ask if today is "movement day," suggesting that they enjoy the program.

As far as early identification of motor or sensory processing difficulties is concerned, the class provides a setting in which a child identified by teacher as prompting concern can be observed by the leader for possible problems or vice versa. Generally, when both the leader and classroom teacher are concerned about a child's skills, parents are likely to follow through on recommendations for referral for a formal evaluation. Referrals might be for further medical follow up, an occupational therapy evaluation or speech and language evaluations. This collaboration seems to lend credibility to teacher comments in conferences with parents.

APPLICABILITY TO OTHER PROGRAMS

Some of the Movement Is Fun activities have now been used with other groups of preschool children, i.e., in therapy sessions with small groups. In addition, the program was adapted for use with a classroom of orthopedically handicapped children who seemed to greatly enjoy the freedom of moving as they wanted to move rather than in the prescribed manner in usual therapy. Finally, some of the program music has been incorporated in individual therapy sessions to facilitate and observe auditory-motor skills. Other applications by therapist are undoubtedly possible. Small groups of visually impaired children, for example, may benefit from the spatial concepts and free movement of such a program.

CONCLUSION

A movement program based on sensory integration theory, incorporating movement education concepts, was developed and has been used for four years in one preschool. Currently, MIF has been added to six preschools in the Kansas City area, reaching approximately 500 children, ages 3-5. The activity involved seems to be fun for children. Potentially, it enhances normal growth and development and provides an opportunity for early identification of sensory motor problems. In addition, such a program is also applicable to dysfunctioning persons. One of the greatest benefits to therapists leading the program, however, is that the opportunity to work with and observe normal children enhances their assessment and treatment skills. Controlled research studies to determine benefits of the program need to be devised and conducted.

REFERENCES

1. Ayres, AJ: *Sensory Integration and Learning Disorders*. Western Psychological Services, 1972

2. Curtis, SR: *The Joy of Movement in Early Education*. New York: Teachers College, Columbia University, 1979

3. Gensemer, R: *Movement Education*. Washington, D.C.: National Education Association, 1979

4. Ayres, AJ: *Sensory Integration and the Child*. Los Angeles: Western Psychological Services, 1979

5. Palmer, H: *Walter the Waltzing Worm*. Freeport, New York: Educational Activities, Inc., 1982

6. Rose, N: *Nothing To Do*. The Children's Record Guild

7. Palmer, H: *Getting To Know Myself*. Freeport, New York: Educational Activities, Inc., 1972

8. Stallman, L and Susser, B: *Pre-Square Dance*. Roslyn, New York: Educational Systems, Inc., 1971

Sensory Integrative Dysfunction: Parental Participation in the Child's Therapy Program

Janet S. Hamill, MOT, OTR/L

SUMMARY. Parental participation in the occupational therapy program for the child with sensory integrative dysfunction may significantly improve the achievement of therapy goals, as well as adaptive behaviors within the home. An individual plan for effective parent involvement is developed with consideration given to levels of parent/child interaction and to the parents' ability to accept their child's difficulties. Purposes of parental participation are outlined in conjunction with an existing model for evaluation and intervention. A case presentation is presented which illustrates optimal parental involvement and the resulting positive outcomes.

The child with sensory integrative dysfunction is often described by his parents as being distractible, having a short attention span, and displaying erratic or inappropriate behavior. Parents often observe that their child is delayed in self care independence, cannot follow instructions or complete tasks, has problems with changes in routine and sleeping, and may display maladaptive play behavior. For these children, the goal of occupational therapy is to improve adaptive responses to both home and school environments, thereby facilitating learning and more appropriate behavior.[1] As a result of occupational therapy intervention for sensory integrative dysfunc-

Janet S. Hamill is an occupational therapist at the Elizabethtown Hospital and Rehabilitation Center, The Pennsylvania State University, Elizabethtown, PA.

Acknowledgements: Appreciation is extended to John, David, and Teresa, and to their parents who have provided a source of inspiration for this article. The author also wishes to thank Geoffrey Hamill for his support.

This article appears jointly in *Sensory Integrative Approaches in Occupational Therapy* (The Haworth Press, 1987) and *Occupational Therapy in Health Care*, Volume 4, Number 2 (Summer 1987).

47

tion, there should be an improvement in the child's ability to function at home.

This author has worked as an occupational therapist in a variety of settings, including public and private schools, residential and day facilities, clinics and hospitals. In each of these places a direct relationship was recognized between the degree of parental participation in their child's therapy program and the child's achievements. Greater parental involvement and understanding of occupational therapy for sensory integrative disorders resulted in remarkable improvement in the child's response to therapy and in behavior at home.

The current literature is limited in its study of the parents' role in their child's occupational therapy program.[2] In her book, *Sensory Integration and the Child*, Ayres outlines the crucial role parents have in facilitating their child's progress.[1] Parents of children with sensory integrative dysfunction should: (1) recognize and understand their child's needs; (2) help to develop their child's self esteem; (3) control the environment at home; (4) help their child learn how to play, and (5) seek professional help.

This article presents factors to consider when determining appropriate levels of parental participation and describes a positive role for parents in therapy. The article also provides information regarding the practical application of occupational therapy home programs as an adjunct to therapy. A case presentation is included to illustrate how dramatic gains in therapy goals may be associated with optimal parent participation in the child's therapy program.

CONSIDERATIONS FOR PARENT PARTICIPATION

As the child begins therapy, an early consideration should be to determine how best to involve the parents. It is important to assess how the parents spontaneously interact with their child, and the degree to which they have come to accept their child's disability.

Bromwich discusses the interaction between parent and infant in terms of a hierarchial model, the Parent Behavior Progression.[3] The six levels of the Behavior Progression are briefly described here as follows:

Level I: The parent enjoys her infant.
Level II: The parent is a sensitive observer of her in-

fant, reads his behavioral cues accurately and is responsive to them.

Level III: The parent engages in a quality of interaction with her infant that is mutually satisfying and that provides opportunity for the development of attachment.

Level IV: The parent demonstrates an awareness of materials, activities, and experiences suitable for her infant's current stage of development.

Level V: The parent initiates new play activities and experiences based on principles that she has internalized from her own experiences, or on the same principles as activities suggested to or modeled for her.

Level VI: The parent independently generates a wide range of developmentally appropriate activities and experiences, interesting to the infant, in familiar and in new situations, and at new levels of the infant's development.

Bromwich has observed that an infant who does not respond to normal parenting behaviors such as holding, stroking or rocking may cause the parent to withdraw from her infant, resulting in a less rewarding interaction. Infants and children with sensory integrative dysfunction may not respond normally to typical parenting behaviors. As a result, a stressful environment is created between parent and infant, fostering inadequate development of the Behavior Progression.

The scheme of the Parent Behavior Progression can be easily adapted for relevance to parents of preschool and school age children with sensory integrative dysfunction. The parents' achievement of normal levels of the Behavior Progression is important for developing a positive outcome to parental participation in their child's occupational therapy program. In this author's experience, the traditional home program of therapy activities is normally effective only when parents achieve levels V or VI of the Behavior Progression. When these levels are not achieved or when gaps occur, the effectiveness of the home program may be severely reduced. For example, it is important for the parents to be able to interpret and understand their child's cues and behavioral responses in order to conduct an effective and therapeutic home program activity, and to give appropriate feedback on the effectiveness of these activities to their therapist.

It follows from the work of Bromwich that an important role of the clinician is to help parents achieve optimal levels of the Behavior Progression and to fill in any gaps, thereby facilitating a positive parent/child interaction and providing an environment conducive to learning. Ayres writes that sensory integrative treatment activities must be motivating or fun for the child in order to promote maximal integration.[1] The therapist can promote positive parent/child interaction through carefully designed home program activities; a mutually fulfilling interaction will create a satisfying experience for the child, and will permit maximal integration to occur.

Another critical factor for successful parent/child interaction relates to the parent's acceptance of their child's disability. Most parents come to accept their child's disability after passing through attitudinal stages related to mourning.[4] Each stage of denial, depression, guilt, anger, bargaining and acceptance will affect the relationship established between the occupational therapist and the parents, as well as between the parents and their child. Parents who can accept their child's sensory integrative dysfunction may participate more effectively in the therapy program, while parents who have not reached this final stage may need support. Empathy for the parents' feelings is essential, as well as clear communication and well defined therapy goals.

PARENT PARTICIPATION: THE ELIZABETHTOWN HOSPITAL AND REHABILITATION CENTER PROGRAM

A child with sensory integrative or learning problems who is referred to Elizabethtown Hospital and Rehabilitation Center receives a complete occupational therapy evaluation. Assessment may include the following: Southern California Sensory Integration Tests,[5] Southern California Postrotary Nystagmus Test,[6] Miller Assessment for Preschoolers,[7] DeGangi-Berk Test of Sensory Integration,[8] Harris-Goodenough Draw-a-Person Test,[9] Test of Visual-Motor Integration,[10] Motor-Free Test of Visual Perception,[11] Test of Hand Dominance,[12] Developmental Programming for Infants and Young Children: Assessment,[13] and clinical observations.

When the child arrives, the parent is asked to complete a questionnaire addressing topics of sensory history, behaviors associated with sensory integrative dysfunction, self care skills, and fine motor skills.[14] A team evaluation of psychological, educational, physical therapy, speech and language, medical or psychiatric assessment is provided according to each child's needs. Evaluation results are presented by the team at a parent conference. A discussion of the child's sensory integrative strengths and weaknesses is often presented by the occupational therapist, using a simplified flow chart.

Once therapy sessions are scheduled, parents are expected to observe or participate when possible. Using the Behavior Progression described earlier, the therapist identifies the level of parent-child interaction based on spontaneous parent-child interactive behaviors, parental report of situations at home and other team members' observations. The amount and type of participation is determined by these affective parameters, as well as the parent's readiness and willingness to participate. In some cases, it is prudent for the parent to not be present initially. For example, should the child have difficulty separating from his mother, she may need to leave the therapy room in order for him to function independently and to establish rapport with the therapist. If the situation permits, the parents are encouraged to watch the therapy session through a oneway mirror. In most cases, however, the parents either observe therapy in the same room or actively participate in therapy activities. It is important that a few minutes be reserved to discuss each day's session, parent concerns, and the home program. When parents cannot be present during therapy sessions, occasional sessions may be videotaped for later viewing.

Initially, the home program consists of one or two suggestions to accomplish some of the parent's immediate concerns (i.e., dressing or self-feeding issues). If these goals are accomplished and the parents are ready for more suggestions, recommendations should begin to focus on structuring the home environment and teaching developmentally appropriate skills to the child. Therapy activities are given to the family only when the above recommendations are followed through successfully. It is emphasized that the home program is an adjunct to regular therapy and that it is monitored and modified weekly.

PURPOSE OF PARENT PARTICIPATION

Parent participation serves several purposes, and six major ones are identified here. *First*, the parents' emotions are supported. It is important for the parents to voice their concerns to the therapist who can then use this opportunity to help them recognize their own attitudes and feelings.[4] Positive parent/child interaction can be modeled by the therapist, and enjoyable sensory experiences (e.g., backrubs before bed, movement activities, or tactile games) set up for parent and child to engage in together.

Second, parent participation will also facilitate better understanding of the child's diagnosis. Parent conferences at regular intervals, as well as brief discussions at the close of each therapy session are essential. As parents observe therapy, they will begin to recognize their child's specific strengths and weaknesses as they relate to therapy goals and activities.

The *third* purpose of parent participation is to help them learn appropriate expectations for their child. Parents can learn to "see with a therapist's eye" as they observe each therapy session and discuss daily progress with the therapist. In this way, the therapist can then guide the parents in setting realistic expectations for behavior and performance expected at home.

The *fourth* purpose of parent involvement is to assist parents in creating a home environment where their child feels secure, competent, and able to organize himself, thereby promoting maximum integration. The child's disorganization is a reflection of his unstable nervous system as it attempts to cope with his constantly changing world. By providing external stability, or structure for their child, parents allow their child to interact adaptively with his environment. In her book, *Learning Disability: A Family Affair*, Osman notes the unique problems of parents with learning disabled children.[15] These children often have a disorganizing effect on the entire family, resulting in spiraling chaos. A more stable situation can usually be created for the whole family by simple changes within the household. The occupational therapist's role is to assess the impact of the daily living activities on the child and the family, and to suggest appropriate changes. The structure that the therapist recommends should be consistent with the child's sensory integrative needs and behavioral abilities. For example, one family was given ideas for creating a special play corner to help their child play more adaptively with her toys and attend for longer periods. Calming tactile input such as a beanbag chair and large pillows, reduced visual distraction, and a white noise tape helped her to focus on the selected activity. Another family removed all distractions from their bathroom and placed a sequenced list on the door to help their son emerge from the bathroom independently with his hands dried and his pants pulled up. In another situation, the parents of a bright five year old provided him with proprioceptive and deep tactile activities prior to dressing in the morning. These activities helped prepare his system to respond to the difficult task of dressing, and minimized his tactile defensiveness as his mother assisted him. A sticker chart helped reinforce his independent skills. Other general ideas for developing structure involve arranging the daily routine so it meets the sensory integrative needs of the child, providing a specific place for items that are easily lost, creating picture or word lists to cue each step in the difficult sequence of a task, and using a timer to help the child deal with time constraints. The child can function more adaptively and independently when appropriate structure is provided.

The *final purpose* of parent participation in therapy is to guide the parents in teaching adaptive play behaviors and self care skills to their child. Parents often need to learn how to structure the play environment so that play experiences will meet their child's needs. Suggestions given by this therapist focus on assisting parents in selecting toys that will meet the child's sensory needs: Hippity Hop, Sit'n Spin, Flying Turtle, scooter boards, or punching dolls are recommended with the individual child's needs in mind. Parents need to recognize that their child may require assistance to organize his play space, and that only a few toys should be put out at one time in order to facilitate his interaction with them. Ayres recommends providing situations that will stimulate the child's inner drive, recognizing that he will usually direct his own sensory needs in adaptive play.[1]

It is generally recognized that a primary place of learning is in the home and that parents are responsible for teaching their children many skills that are important for normal development. Parents with a "clumsy" child may need information regarding appropriate self care skills to work on, and successful approaches to each task. During therapy sessions for these children, this therapist spends some time on functional skills such as lacing, spreading peanut butter, pouring a drink, feeding, or cutting. Parents are often encouraged to work on these activities at home because they are not a major focus of the therapy session. Parents can benefit from learning how to analyze an activity from a sensory-motor view and recognizing their child's responses to such activities. Home program activities are monitored on a weekly basis to encourage positive parent involvement and success for the child.

As the four or five year old becomes independent with basic self care skills, the family is encouraged to begin initiating responsibility for household chores, while taking into account their child's sensory-motor needs and abilities. A child with poor somatosensory processing and dyspraxia may benefit from simple cooking activities with clearly sequenced recipes that involve increased tactile/proprioceptive input. Another child may assist with folding laundry, an activity that will help him learn concepts of directionality, form and space. A task of carrying the laundry or emptying wastebaskets will provide extra proprioceptive input and may facilitate successful completion for a child who has difficulty staying on task while navigating through the house. A check list or sticker chart may help ensure daily success.

CASE PRESENTATION

John is a five year, nine month old boy who lives at home with his parents and two brothers, aged three and seven years. John's prenatal and perinatal history were normal. His mother describes him as a pleasant infant who gained weight slowly; he seemed weaker than his brothers, and developed gross motor skills more slowly. John's early medical history is significant for chronic otitis media between one and two years of age. A hearing loss was detected when John was four and a half years old, necessitating the placement of tympanostomy tubes and an adenoidectomy. Subsequently, his hearing has been normal. John was enrolled in a part-time special education preschool program for eight months; his services were recently reduced to individual sessions lasting one hour per week.

John received a multidisciplinary evaluation at Elizabethtown Hospital and Rehabilitation Center when he was almost five years old. Both parents were present throughout the evaluation and for the parent conference. Their suspicions were confirmed for the first time: John had low-average intelligence, accompanied by motor delays and probable sensory integrative dysfunction. He was "at risk" for learning disabilities. Occupational therapy was recommended at a frequency of one session per week.

Standardized and formal occupational therapy assessments could not be administered initially; John refused to comply with testing because he "was afraid of failing." After six weeks of therapy, John was given the Miller Assessment for Preschoolers,[7] the Southern California Postrotary Nystagmus Test,[6] and clinical observations.[16] (See Table 1 for results.) Results indicated significant vestibular and kinesthetic processing problems associated with low muscle tone, delayed integration of primitive neck reflexes, and inadequate postural and ocular control. Bilateral integration was poorly developed, and was accompanied by an inability to cross body midline. There was no clearly established hand dominance. John appeared dyspraxic, with difficulties in both planning and executing non-habitual skilled movements.

On the parent questionnaire, only 15 of 89 responses were considered adaptive behaviors or normal responses.[14] Immediate parent concerns focused on John's constant destructive play behavior and his difficulty settling down to sleep at night. His lack of judgment and physical safety were also of concern. John's mother reported that he could not dress himself independently. At mealtimes he frequently fell out of his chair and often ate with his fingers because utensils were too difficult to use. John frequently spilled his milk and food, creating a mess on the floor at every meal. John's parents described winter as a particularly difficult time for him. It appears

TABLE 1. Scores from John's evaluation

Miller Assessment for Preschoolers (Percentile Scores)		
	Original	Follow-up
Total Score:	3%	7%
Performance Indices		
Foundations:	5%	31%
Coordination:	11%	4%
Verbal:	10%	99%
Non-Verbal:	30%	53%
Complex Tasks:	4%	4%

Southern California Postrotary Nystagmus Test (Standard Deviations)				
	Original		Follow-up	
	Raw Score	S.D.	Raw Score	S.D
Total Score:		below		
	0	-2.6	25	+0.7

that the reduced amount of vestibular and proprioceptive input that John received indoors caused him to become progressively "wound up" and disorganized, causing a multitude of stresses within the family.

Therapy goals focused on John's ability to integrate vestibular and kinesthetic sensory input, while forming a foundation for improved bilateral integration, praxis, postural and ocular reactions. Sensory integration treatment principles provided the theoretical framework for therapy activities.

John's mother attended each therapy session, and his father observed once. Both parents initially demonstrated an acceptance of John's difficulties as well as interactions consistent with Level V of the Behavior Progression described earlier. They sought out reading materials to further their understanding of John's sensory integrative dysfunction. John's mother observed treatment sessions, and gradually began to participate in activities when requested by the therapist. She quickly developed unusually clear insight regarding John's sensory needs and his responses, in therapy and at home.

Self care and prewriting activities were frequently scheduled for the latter part of each session, emphasizing tasks relevant to John at home. John's mother was able to learn from the therapist's modeling and expanded on the activities at home. After each session, John's progress was briefly reviewed with his mother to help her understand his responses. The home program was informally monitored, and sensory-motor games were occasionally loaned.

John's first home program focused on the parents' primary concerns of his play and sleep behaviors. Suggestions for play involved selecting a few appropriate toys and removing breakable items from the area. John's mother found that he fell asleep more easily when a consistent bedtime routine was followed and distracting toys were removed from his bedside; a soothing backrub helped him calm more easily. John's parents appeared ready for more suggestions to structure the environment; independently they began to initiate many appropriate changes at home and demonstrated interactions consistent with Level VI of the Behavior Progression.

Consistent daily routines and clearly defined limits helped provide structure. A daily list on the refrigerator of things to do has helped John plan his day and realize his accomplishments. At mealtimes, John was separated from his brothers to reduce the distractions and minimize friction. John used a heavy ceramic mug and junior spoon and fork to help give increased sensory feedback; these improved his feeding skills. A plastic sheet on the floor helped reduce parental stress over spills. Appropriate seating with a seat belt or Dycem Pad was recommended to provide more stability during feeding and fine motor activities.

Home program recommendations were given for such things as: dressing, pouring, and spreading with a knife. Difficult tasks were broken down into components that John could successfully master. John's parents demonstrated both the willingness and capability to follow through with selected therapy activities at home as an adjunct to the therapy program. They constructed a scooter board and bolster swing and created a safe, padded area to use the equipment. John's parents observed that controlled amounts of vestibular input in the form of specific activities had a broad effect in helping John organize himself for more adaptive behavior at home. Vestibular and proprioceptive activities were found to help John prepare his system for difficult fine motor tasks when performed prior to visual-motor activities.

In the past eight months, John has made significant gains, as demonstrated by his test results (see Table 1). The clinical observations revealed normal postural mechanisms and antigravity movement components, improved ocular control, bilateral integration, and ability to cross midline.

Improvements at home were reflected in a dramatically higher score of adaptive behaviors as measured by a follow-up parent questionnaire (57 out of 89 responses). John's parents report that he demonstrates much better judgment and is physically safe in most situations. He sits independently in his chair at mealtime, and is managing utensils with more skill. John has become independent with dressing. He can now play constructively with peers and often takes initiative to put things away. John is contributing to daily chores by emptying the wastebaskets and carrying the laundry.

Cognitive re-evaluation by the psychologist indicated intelligence slightly above average. Achievement test scores were above age expectation; thus, John is not presently classified as "learning disabled." John will attend a regular kindergarten and will receive resource help with handwriting and fine motor skills.

In summary, John made significant gains in sensory integrative and cognitive function, as well as remarkable improvements in his adaptive behavior in therapy and at home. These results are probably due to early therapeutic intervention and optimal participation by John's parents in the therapy program. John's parents felt the input they received from the occupational therapist was a pivotal factor related to John's improvement at home. Though John's education program may also have contributed to his gains, it should be noted that his preschool program began seven months before the original test data and was greatly curtailed four months later.

CONCLUSION

Parental participation in the child's therapy program should be considered when therapy begins and should be based on the parent's readiness and the child's needs.

A number of benefits are derived when the parents observe or participate in therapy, and when they follow through with recommendations at home. Parental participation will improve the child's gains in therapy, as well as his function at home.

REFERENCES

    1. Ayres AJ: *Sensory Integration and the Child*. Los Angeles: Western Psychological Services, 1983

    2. Friedman: A program for parents of children with sensory integration dysfunction. *AJOT* 36: 9,1982, p. 586-589

    3. Bromwich RM: *Working with Parents and Infants: An Interactional Approach*, Baltimore University Park Press, 1981, p. 55-57

    4. Hanft B: *Managing an Early Intervention Program*. University Affiliated Program: University of South Carolina, Winthrop College, 1980

    5. Ayres AJ: *Southern California Sensory Integration Tests*, Los Angeles: Western Psychological Services, 1972

    6. Ayres AJ: *Southern California Postrotary Nystagmus Test*, Los Angeles: Western Psychological Services, 1972

    7. Miller L: *Miller Assessment for Preschoolers*, Littleton, CO: The Foundation for Knowledge in Development, 1982

    8. DeGangi G, Berk R: *DeGangi-Berk Test of Sensory Integration*, Los Angeles: Western Psychological Services, 1983

    9. Harris D: *Children's Drawings as Measures of Intellectual Maturity*. New York: Harcourt Brace Jovanovich, Inc. 1963

    10. Beery K: *Developmental Test of Visual-Motor Integration*, Cleveland, OH: Modern Curriculum Press, 1982

    11. Colarusso R, Hammill D: *Motor-Free Visual Perception Test*. Novato, CA: Academic Therapy Publications, 1972

    12. Knickerbocker BM: *A Holistic Approach to the Treatment of Learning Disorders*. Thorofare, NJ: Charles B Slack, Inc., 1980

13. Rogers S, D'Eugenio D: *Developmental Programming for Infants and Young Children: Assessments and Application*. Ann Arbor, MI: University of Michigan Press, 1981

14. Hamill J: *Elizabethtown Hospital and Rehabilitation Center Parent Questionnaire*. Elizabethtown, PA: unpublished assessment

15. Osman B: *Learning Disability: A Family Affair*. New York: Warner Books Edition, 1979

16. Dunn W: *A Guide to Testing Clinical Observations in Kindergartners*. Rockville, MD: American Occupational Therapy Association, Inc., 1981

Sensory Integration and Play Behavior: A Case Study of the Effectiveness of Occupational Therapy Using Sensory Integrative Techniques

Roseann C. Schaaf, MEd, OTR/L
Susan Cook Merrill, MA, OTR/L
Nancy Kinsella, OTR/L

SUMMARY. This paper presents a case study describing a developmentally delayed child and examines the changes in environmental interactions that occurred during a study period in occupational therapy in which sensory integration (SI) techniques were applied. Its purpose is to discuss the use of play observation as a means of measuring change in individuals involved in SI treatment and to demonstrate the relevance of qualitative research methodologies to the collection of data on play behavior. The study is a first step in a process of developing methods to evaluate the effectiveness of SI treatment in occupational therapy through collecting qualitative data on play and other behavioral measures of environmental interactions.

Acknowledgements: The authors wish to thank KenCrest Centers of Philadelphia for the use of their facility to conduct this study, and Elizabeth DePoy, MSW, OTR/L for her rigorous editorial assistance and constant encouragement.

Roseann C. Schaaf and Susan Cook Merrill are faculty members in the Department of Occupational Therapy, Thomas Jefferson University, Philadelphia, PA. In addition, Ms. Schaaf is in private practice with a pediatric specialty; Ms. Merrill is a consultant to the Occupational Therapy Department, Hahneman University Hospital. Nancy Kinsella, a recent graduate of TJU, is an occupational therapist at KenCrest Centers, Philadelphia.

This article appears jointly in *Sensory Integrative Approaches in Occupational Therapy* (The Haworth Press, 1987) and *Occupational Therapy in Health Care*, Volume 4, Number 2 (Summer 1987).

The need to evaluate the effectiveness of occupational therapy intervention using sensory integrative (SI) techniques has been a frequent research topic in the profession.[1,2,3] Studies which have examined the usefulness of SI treatment have largely relied on traditional, quantitative research methods.[4-9] The purposes of this paper are to present a case study describing a developmentally delayed child and to examine the changes in his interactions with his environment that occurred during an eight week period during occupational therapy using SI methods. Further the use of play observation as a qualitative research method for measuring change will be examined and evaluated as a relevant strategy for collecting data on play behavior.

In the case study a theoretical framework which combines sensory integration and occupational behavior is used because both theories emphasize the importance of play as a reflection of child development and as a major role in childhood.[10,11,12] Each framework views play as a behavior which reflects the individual's ability to interact with his environment in a competent manner. Dysfunction in environmental interactions due to faulty sensory integration, poor motivation or locus of control will result in play dysfunction.[13] Writings of both Ayres and Reilly[10-12] reflect the importance of childhood play as a foundation for later learning ability and environmental interactions.[11,12]

Central to SI theory is the premise that treatment will affect an individual's ability to interact adaptively within the environment.[11] Ayres terms these interactions "adaptive responses" dependent upon and leading to adequate sensory integration and subsequent nervous system maturation.[10,11] SI theory maintains that play behavior is related to sensory integration and that poor sensory integration will adversely affect play behavior. In turn, poor play behavior will impede the normal sensory integrative process.[13] By examining an individual's adaptive responses, clues can be obtained about the ability of the nervous system to process and integrate environmental stimuli. Treatment is aimed at enhancing the nervous system's ability to process and organize information so an individual can interact with his environment in an efficacious manner.[6]

Ayres concentrates on the motivational aspect of play behavior as indicative of neural functioning. She believes that play reflects a child's neuromotor system and that difficulty in integrating and processing sensory information will result in play dysfunction.[11] A child with normal sensory integrative processes will seek appropriate play experiences to further growth and development. On the other hand, a child with dysfunction in sensory integration abilities will often avoid or not know how to engage in normal, growth-perpetuating play experiences. A dysfunctional child may seek ways to fulfill the intrinsic need for environmental and sensory input, but these ways may be maladaptive in nature.

The view of play behavior as an indicator of a child's ability to process and integrate environmental stimuli for purposeful behavior is not unique to SI theory.[12,14-16] Reilly,[12] using a theoretical approach which draws heavily from both Piaget[14] and White,[15] describes play as neurogenic and as having social and cultural importance in childhood as the child prepares and rehearses for later adult roles. She emphasizes that play is experiential learning and she believes that the direct experience derived from play activities facilitates the learning process more quickly than passive vicarious experiences. Reilly uses White's[15] depiction of play as a hierarchy which begins with intrinsic urges and motivation to explore the environment and progresses to more extrinsic factors. She classifies three levels of play: exploration behavior/play, competence behavior/play and achievement behavior/play.

Thus this case draws from the perspective on play of both Ayres and Reilly as it examines the changes in a child's interactions with the environment, as measured by play behavior, that occur during the course of a period of occupational therapy using SI techniques.

METHODOLOGY

Case study and qualitative research methodologies which facilitate a process whereby specific treatment interventions could be examined without intruding on the client's treatment regime, were used in this study. Qualitative research methods involve the collection of descriptive data to which numbers cannot productively be applied.[17-20] Many forms of qualitative research exist including ethnography and life history.[17] Methods of data collection include observation, participation and structured and semistructured interviews. Analysis of data usually involves summarizing in narrative form.[19] The reader is referred to several texts for further information on these methods.[18-21] The relationship between the underlying values and assumptions of occupational therapy and principles of qualitative methods have been explored in recent literature.[1,21-26]

In an attempt to gather as much information as possible about the subject's environmental interactions and to verify the accuracy of the data, four sources of data collection were used: a *teacher questionnaire* (Table 1), a 10 minute *free play observation* when the subject was with other children in the class and when various preschool play activities were available, *occupational therapy treat-*

TABLE I

EXAMPLE OF TEACHER PLAY QUESTIONNAIRE

Date _____ Child's Name _____ Rater _____

Please answer the following questions to the best of your knowledge. The major purpose of this questionnaire is to monitor any significant changes in your child's play behaviors which may be related to improved ability to interact within the environment. We are attempting to determine if any changes in the child's behavior may be related to therapeutic intervention. THANK YOU.

1. What does your child do with his/her unstructured (free play) time?

    1a. Is this a change from what he/she usually does? If so, how is it different?

2. What has been your child's favorite toy or activity lately?

    2a. Describe how your child plays with this toy/activity.

3. How did your child respond to changes in routine this week?

4. Have you noticed any specific changes in your child this week? If so, are they attributable to anything in particular?

5. Has there been a significant increase or decrease in any of the following? (If so please elaborate):
    Interactions with peers and family members?

    Independence in dressing, feeding or play?

    Dependency on teacher or parent(s)?

    Mood changes?

    Verbalizations?

6. Has there been an increase or decrease in activity level during this week?

7. Has there been any increase or decrease in behaviors, such as self-stimulating behaviors, temper tantrums, play, frustration tolerance, etc.? If so, when do you notice these behaviors? Is there anything that seems to trigger such behaviors?

8. Has there been an increase or decrease in sensitivity to stimuli, such as tactile stimuli, food, clothing, noise, etc.? If so, please elaborate.

PLEASE ADD ANY OTHER COMMENTS THAT MAY BE USEFUL. THANK YOU!

(Schaaf & Merrill, 1985)

ment records and *The Davis Hyperactivity Scale.*[27] The teacher questionnaire solicits comment on toys and activities that the subject engages in during free play in the classroom in a given week, and elaboration on how the subject functions in those activities. The questionnaire focuses on the quality of the subject's playful interactions and his behavior during play. Questions regarding the subject's language, social interactions, activity level, level of independence or dependence and emotional status are also included.

The occupational therapist who treats the subject collected data on play by observing a 10 minute free play session (described above) one time per week. These data consisted of records of behavior, play, object relations, language and social interactions during the period. Table 2 shows an example of the form used for this method of data collection. In addition, as a third source, weekly progress notes from occupational therapy, elaborating on activities used in and responses to treatment, were used. Finally, the subject's activity level and distractability were assessed by the teacher during a baseline period and again at the end of treatment using the Davids Hyperactivity Scale. Parents were also requested to observe and record the subject's behavior and activity at home using the play questionnaire, but there was minimal return on this request. Data were collected for two baseline periods (two weeks) and eight treatment periods (8 weeks).

THE CASE

RS is a 4 year old male diagnosed as developmentally delayed in all areas of development. At the time of occupational therapy evaluation, in February 1986, he was 4 years, 0 months old and functioning at an approximately 12 to 15 month level in all areas of performance. RS had received speech therapy since June 1985 and was on no medication during the study. He is the product of a pregnancy complicated by hypoglycemia, hypothyroidism and an automobile accident three weeks prior to his delivery. Early developmental history indicated slow acquisition of motor skills; neurological examination revealed increased activity level, low frustration tolerance and head banging; the audiologist found adequate auditory sensitivity for speech.

The boy lived with his mother, grandmother and grandfather and visits his father on occasional weekends. He has attended nursery

TABLE 2

EXAMPLE OF WORKSHEET FOR DATA COLLECTION OF PLAY OBSERVATION

Play Observation

Date of Observation_____Child's Name _____

Data Collector_____Area_____

TIME	TOY	INTERACTION WITH TOY	SOCIAL/LANGUAGE	COMMENTS

school since one and one-half years of age and is presently enrolled in a 5 day per week, federally funded, private non-profit, early intervention program for developmentally delayed preschoolers. At the time of the study, in addition to his preschool classroom program and speech therapy, RS was receiving occupational therapy one time per week. Occupational therapy consultation was available to classroom teachers on an ongoing basis. Occupational therapy developmental and observational evaluation, completed 3 months prior to the study, describes RS as extremely distractable during evaluation with particular sensitivity to auditory stimulation. He had difficulty with a structured evaluation and therefore was given the opportunity for a less structured developmental and observational evaluation when he appeared more relaxed and performed more competently.

The evaluation revealed that RS is delayed in all areas of development and his performance and behavior suggest sensory integrative dysfunction as part of his disability. Motor planning difficulties were evident; he demonstrated emotional lability, low frustration tolerance, high activity level and distractability, particularly to auditory stimuli. He was noted to seek and enjoy vestibular and proprioceptive activities. Additional difficulties displayed during the initial treatment session include distractability to the point of often leaving an activity to lie on the floor for no apparent reason one to three times during the 45 minute session. (This behavior was also observed in the classroom.) He chose, and tolerated for only 10-45 seconds, vestibular and proprioceptive activities; demonstrated difficulty in motor planning; for example, in getting on and off equipment he often needed physical assistance. His communication attempts were incoherent or gestural more than 50 percent of the time. He was dependent in dressing and undressing, inconsistent with zipping and unzipping, was not toilet trained, and was unable to dry his hands or wipe his nose. During the initial treatment sessions he appeared fearful, sad and tense; his jaw was often clenched in a fearful grimace and he was noted to grind his teeth frequently. He often demonstrated aggressive behaviors such as hitting and spitting.

The treatment plan for RS included goals to improve sensory integrative functioning, particularly of tactile, proprioceptive and vestibular systems; improve muscle tone, righting and equilibrium reactions; improve motor planning; facilitate gross and fine motor skills; enhance visual perceptual skills and improve independence in dressing.

DATA ANALYSIS

Data were reviewed by three occupational therapists. Two, each with ten years of clinical experience, are certified to administer the Southern California Sensory Integration Tests. The third reviewer was the therapist directly involved in treating the child under the supervision of the other two, who collected data by play observation. Each therapist reviewed all data independently after which group meetings were held to discuss and arrive at consensus on patterns and trends of behavior seen and to develop categories of behavior to be monitored. For example, it was felt by the three that interaction/manipulation with objects was a category of behavior demonstrated in RS's play data, so progression of this behavior was reviewed.

In discussing the trends of behaviors revealed from the data, the presence of the therapist who actually observed RS was crucial. She was able to substantiate or negate the observations based on having seen the actual play activity. For example, if the data stated that the child was sitting alone and rocking in a boat, the therapist could qualify if this play activity appeared to be of a self-stimulating nature or a playful interaction. Such information was vital and added to the validity of the interpretation process. Four groups of data were analyzed in this manner: the play observations made by the therapist, the play observation/questionnaire completed by the teacher; the occupational therapy records/notes and the scores of the Davids Hyperactivity Scale.

RESULTS

Review of data yielded a number of categories of behavior. These are listed in Table 3. Of those, four, listed below, were chosen for analysis because in all of them RS showed change in *each* of the four groups of data. Since others of the behavior categories did not show identifiable trends in *all* forms of data collection, comments made about them are more speculative. However, those categories

TABLE 3

CATEGORIES OF BEHAVIOR DELINEATED FROM QUALITATIVE REVIEW OF DATA

Interactions/manipulations with objects

Verbalizations: intelligibility and frequency of utterances

Interactions with others

Sensory exploration of environment

Bruxism (teeth grinding)

Tolerance of vestibular input

Tolerance of environment (before withdrawing)

Strategies for dealing with frustration

Transition time from one activity to another

Time spent on one activity

Activity level

of behavior that showed consistent patterns of change throughout the data are considered to be important observations upon which statements of RS's behavior can be made. They are:

Interactions/manipulations of objects
Interactions with others
Tolerance to vestibular/proprioceptive input
Sensory exploration of the environment

Interaction/Manipulation of Objects

In this category RS demonstrated a marked progression during the 8 week treatment period. His behavior evolved from simple dumping/filling play and throwing and/or taking of toys to more mature manipulations of simple toys. For example, in the baseline data RS was observed to dump out blocks from a cylindrical container and then simply put them back in. By the middle of the treatment period, he was beginning to attempt to put two blocks together, watching other children build with blocks, and manipulating other objects in an appropriate manner such as winding a toy radio, banging on a musical instrument in an acceptable way and manipulating a zipper on a doll. This change in object manipulation was noted both in the teacher and therapist play observations as well as in the occupational therapy treatment notes.

Social Interaction

This was another area in which RS demonstrated positive progression. During both baseline and initial treatment periods RS appeared generally unaware of other children in his environment, interacting only in socially unacceptable ways: hitting, biting or taking toys away from others. By the middle of the treatment sequence he was tolerating other individuals in the environment by sitting beside them (first the teacher, then other children) and finally engaging in parallel play with them. During the last play observation he was playing on a bolster at the same time as three other children and was observed playing with a doll appropriately. This change in social interactions was obvious from both the teacher and therapist play observations. In the therapy notes RS was recorded as smiling and laughing more, with less frequent outbursts.

Tolerance to Vestibular/Proprioceptive Stimuli

Baseline play observations and therapy notes verified that RS sought and appeared to enjoy vestibular/proprioceptive toys but his tolerance for them was limited to 10-45 seconds. As the 8 week treatment period progressed, he spent longer amounts of time with such equipment both in free play and in treatment sessions and he used the equipment in a more appropriate manner. For example, he rocked on a bolster with other children and seemed to be pretending it was a ride.

Exploration of the Environment

In the initial data collection period, RS showed limited sensory exploration of his surroundings, except auditorily. For example, in response to auditory stimuli he would stop playing and run toward a door from which a noise was coming, or stop and point to any sound stimuli. He progressed to exploration involving more tactile and vestibular sensations, first by mouthing and sitting on objects and rocking and/or shaking them, and later to exploring tactually with his hands on objects. This more mature sensory exploration concurred with both an increase in tolerance for vestibular/proprioceptive activities and to increased manipulation of objects.

Several other areas of improved behavior were noted in RS during this study period but were not so forcefully shown by the data. Bruxism (teeth grinding) initially demonstrated, diminished steadily over the 8 week period and was noted to be absent in the final weeks. Intelligibility of speech and quality of vocalizations also improved. Therapy records indicated he used fewer gestures more and improved speech and occasionally 3 word sentences. Substantial increases in independence in dressing, toileting and hygiene were also documented in the therapy notes. The therapist and teachers commented that while they did not specifically work on dressing skills with RS, nonetheless by the end of the 8 week treatment program, he was dressing, undressing and toileting himself with minimal assistance. Substantial improvement in motor planning was also evident in therapy notes. By the end of the data collection period RS was able to move on and off of new equipment independently and with more coordinated movements. None of these skills was taught, but still his ability to motor plan and to use them improved.

Other changes, as indicated by therapy notes, include improved ability to follow two-step directions, improved righting and equilibrium reactions, decreased distractibility to auditory stimuli and improved emotional tone. Further, RS appeared more relaxed, less aggressive and seemed to enjoy therapy sessions.

In summary, qualitative analysis of the data revealed changes in specific types of behaviors and interactions with the environment. The most notable changes were in the areas of interactions with objects and people, tolerance for vestibular/proprioceptive stimuli and sensory exploration of the environment. Other changes were noted in one or more forms of data, however, statements about these changes are more speculative since they were not documented in all four forms of data collection. Failure of these behavioral changes to appear in all forms of data collection may be the result of decreased sensitivity of the methods used to collect the data, lack of realization by the recorder that the behaviors were significant and relevant for comment or simply, lack of noticeable change in them.

DISCUSSION/IMPLICATIONS

This study represents the first step in a process of developing a coherent methodology for evaluating by observation the effectiveness of sensory integration procedures in occupational therapy. While case study and qualitative methods cannot determine causality, they proved invaluable in this study in documenting change that occurred in one individual during the course of 8 weeks of occupational therapy using SI techniques.

In reviewing some of the most significant changes that were observed in RS, it is noted that several positive changes in behavior occurred at the same time that, with improved ability to process sensory information was noted and documented by therapy notes. For example, an increase in manipulation of objects which was documented in the qualitative data coincided with both increased tolerance to various types of sensory stimuli and improved motor planning as documented by therapy notes. Improved social interactions and decreased aggressive behaviors were documented and coincide with increased tolerance to sensory stimuli in the environment and increased manipulation and interactions with toys. These improvements in environmental interactions, which occurred at the same time gains in occupational therapy using SI techniques were documented, is consistent with a basic theoretical construct of sensory integration, i.e., that improved sensory integration will enhance an individual's ability to respond adaptively to his environment.

Several other positive changes documented in the occupational therapy notes deserve discussion. Fewer aggressive behaviors, more organized behavior and increased independence in self-help skills were shown even though they were not skills specifically addressed in therapy. These changes are consistent with a basic construct of occupational behavior, i.e., that changes in environmental exploration can give rise to a sense of mastery. Such changes also reflect sensory integration theory in that improved nervous system maturation will improve the quality of adaptive responses. Although no statements can be made about the relationship of treatment and the acquisition of skills, this case raises the question of the extent to which occupational therapy using SI techniques affects the acquisition of such skills and behaviors.

Activity level, frustration, self-stimulating behaviors and distractability were all behaviors that did not show any significant trends during the data collection periods. However, both the therapist and the teachers felt that RS did demonstrate subtle improvements in these areas of performance. Whether permanent changes in these behaviors occurred is impossible to comment on at this time; nonetheless, it prompts one to examine the methods/instruments used for data collection and their sensitivity to certain behaviors such as those noted above.

In regard to the instruments used, the informal play observation was the most informative and valuable method as it provided indepth qualitative information about the child's play behavior from which behavioral patterns and characteristics emerged. The play questionnaire was used by both the teacher and the therapist to gather data about RS's play behavior during the school day. Although a potential bias exists since the occupational therapy data collector was aware of the purpose of the study, these two methods of data collection nonetheless appear to have potential as tools for evaluating the effectiveness of occupational therapy using SI techniques. It seems they provide invaluable clues into the child's interactions with his environment and how those may change during the course of treatment. The most important changes that appear to occur as a result of one's sensory integration are those that affect one's occupational performance. In this case, a child's play and the play observation and questionnaire were sensitive to detecting many of these changes. It is unfortunate that the parent data were not returned consistently for this additional input might have provided further valuable information regarding RS's environmental interactions and other changes they observed.

Use of the Davids Hyperactivity Scale did not detect many of the changes in behavior that were documented qualitatively. Although this scale may be useful in quantitatively measuring changes in activity level and attention span over a long period of time, no significant changes were noted in RS during an 8 week treatment program. This could be related to the shortness of the study period. On the other hand, the occupational therapy notes provided valuable qualitative information about RS's behavior, interactions and progress during therapy, and were critical in providing a basis upon which changes in behavior in treatment could be compared to progress seen elsewhere.

CONCLUSION

In addition to introducing potential methods for data collection regarding play behavior, this study has raised several other important questions, the most obvious of which is, "to what extent does occupational therapy using an SI approach affect an individual's interactions with his environment as measured by play behavior?" This differs admittedly from the original question which sparked this study, but one of the purposes of qualitative research is to generate research questions along related lines. Other questions raised by this study include: "how do play and other environmental interactions reflect the integrity of the central nervous system in processing and integrating sensory information?" and "what does the play behavior of other children with conditions similar to RS demonstrate?" Searching for answers to these questions will benefit occupational therapy and add to a growing body of knowledge about human behavior and function.

Observations of the play behavior provided the most consistent and detailed descriptions of changes that occurred in RS's interactions with his environment. Both Reilly[12] and Ayres[11] view play as behavior which reflects an individual's ability to interact with his surroundings in an adaptive manner. This study has begun to examine this theoretical supposition. Further exploration of how one can assess the relationship between SI techniques and play behavior would be extremely valuable to occupational therapy.

REFERENCES

1. Yerxa, EJ: Evaluation versus research: Outcomes or knowledge? *Am J Occup Ther* 38, 407-408, 1984

2. Ottenbacher, K: Sensory integration therapy: Affect or effect. *Am J Occup Ther* 36(9) 571-578, 1982

3. Ottenbacher, K and Short, MA: Publication trends in occupational therapy. *Occup Ther J Res* 2, 80-88, 1982

4. Ayres, AJ: Effect of sensory integrative therapy on the coordination of children with choreoathetoid movements. *Am J Occup Ther* 31(5): 291-293, 1977

5. Ayres, AJ: Improving academic scores through sensory integration. *J Learn Dis* 5, 336-343, 1977

6. Ayres, AJ and Mailloux, Z: Influence of sensory integration procedures on language development. *Am J Occup Ther* 6, 383-390, 1981

7. Ayres, AJ: Learning disabilities and the vestibular system. *J Learn Dis* 11(1), 18-29, 1978

8. Kanter, RM, Kanter, B, and Clark, D: Vestibular stimulation effect on language developmentally retarded children. *Am J Occup Ther* 36(1): 36-41, 1982

9. Ottenbacher, K, Short, MA, and Watson, PJ: The effects of a clinically applied program of vestibular stimulation on the neuromotor performance of children with severe developmental disability. *Phys Occup Ther in Pediat* 1(3), 1-9, 1981

10. Ayres, AJ: *Sensory Integration and Learning Disorders.* Los Angeles, CA: Western Psychological Services, 1972

11. Ayres, AJ: *Sensory Integration and the Child.* Los Angeles, CA: Western Psychological Services, 1979

12. Reilly, M: *Play as Exploratory Learning.* Beverly Hills: Sage Publications, Inc., 1974

13. Lindquist, JE, Mack, W, and Parham, D: A synthesis of occupational behavior and sensory integration concepts in theory and practice, Part 1 and 2. Theoretical Foundations and Clinical Applications. *Am J Occup Ther* 36(6 and 7), 365-374, 433-437, 1982

14. Piaget, J: *Play, Dreams and Imitation in Childhood.* New York: Norton, 1952

15. White, R: Motivation reconsidered: The concept of competence. *Psychological Rev* 66, 10-23, 1959

16. Neville, A, Keilhofner, G, Brasic-Royeen, C: In Kielhofner, G (Ed.): *A Model of Human Occupation: Theory and Application* (pp. 82-98). Baltimore: Williams and Wilkins, 1985

17. Edgerton, RB, and Langness, LL: *Methods and Styles in the Study of Culture.* San Francisco: Chandler and Sharp Publishers, 1974

18. Glaser, BG and Strauss, AL: *The Discovery of Grounded Theory: Strategies for Qualitative Research.* New York: Aldine Publishing Co., 1967

19. Lawless, R, Sutlive, VH, and Zamora, MD: *Fieldwork, The Human Experience.* New York: Gordon and Breach Science Publishers, 1983

20. Patton, MQ: *Qualitative Evaluation Methods.* Beverly Hills: Sage Publications, 1980

21. Kielhofner, G: *An ethnographic study of deinstitutionalized adults: Their community settings and daily life experiences. Occup Ther Res*, 1, 125-143, 1981

22. Kielhofner, G: Qualitative research: Part one: Paradigmatic grounds and issues of reliability and validity. *Occup Ther J Res*, 2, 67-79, 1982

23. Kielhofner, G: Qualitative research: Part two: Methodological approaches and relevance to occupational therapy. *Occup Ther J Res*, 2, 150-164, 1982

24. Merrill, SC: Qualitative methods in occupational therapy research: An application. *Occup Ther J Res*, 5, 209-222, 1985

25. Schmid, J: Qualitative research and occupational therapy. *Amer J Occup Ther* 35, 820-821, 1981

26. Yerxa, EJ; Basic or applied? A "developmental assessment" of occupational therapy reserach in 1981. *Am J Occup Ther* 35, 820-821, 1981

27. Davids, A: An objective instrument for assessing hyperkinesis in children. *J Learn Dis* 4(9), 499-503, 1971

A Sensory-Integrative Approach
to the Education
of the Autistic Child

Lorna Jean King, OTR, FAOTA

SUMMARY. The history and current status of a four year old demonstration school for autistic children in Phoenix, Arizona is described. The curriculum is based on neurodevelopmental, sensory integrative principles as contrasted with operant conditioning models. An interdisciplinary staff integrates communication, daily living, academic and sensorimotor and music components. A neurological frame of reference is described for dealing with self-stimulating and self-abusive behaviors. Awareness of the problems of parents is emphasized.

The Developmental Day School is, to the best of our knowledge, the only state certified school for autistic children in the United States whose administrator is an occupational therapist and whose educational philosophy is based on principles of neurological development.

Located in Phoenix, Arizona, the school is a program of the Center for Neurodevelopmental Studies, a non-profit corporation founded in 1978. The Center provides therapy for persons with a wide spectrum of developmental delays and dysfunctions, but it is the plight of the autistic child that has demanded our special attention.

Lorna Jean King is Director, The Center for Neurodevelopmental Studies, Phoenix, AZ.
This article appears jointly in *Sensory Integrative Approaches in Occupational Therapy* (The Haworth Press, 1987) and *Occupational Therapy in Health Care*, Volume 4, Number 2 (Summer 1987).

77

Autism is a rare syndrome (4 to 5 in 10,000 births), but it is a devastating disability characterized by severe language and communication deficits, lack of normal relatedness, bizarre movement and self stimulating patterns, lack of normal handling of toys and other objects and lack of most normal functional skills. Inability to learn in usual ways results in apparent retardation in many cases, though I.Q. (to the degree it can be measured) can range from genius to severe or profound retardation.

Autism, as described by Kanner in 1943,[1] was thought by him to be a psychiatric condition caused by cold and unloving parents. The prescribed treatment was psychoanalytic, was available to few, and was notably unproductive. By 1968 it was becoming quite clear that autism was, in fact, a neurological disorder described by Ornitz, Ritvo and the U.C.L.A. group of child psychiatrists and pediatric neurologists as a "sensory integrative disorder."[2] Bernard Rimland, PhD, in his 1964 award winning book "*Infantile Autism*,"[3] made a good case for the reticular activating system as the site of damage in autism. The Doctors Wing[4] in England had investigated in detail the sensory abnormalities of autistic children, who seemed unable to process distance receptors (vision and hearing) while relying primarily on olfaction and touch. Vestibular system abnormalities had been investigated by Loretta Bender,[5] Barbara Fish[6] and others, and, in fact, had been an important focus of the U.C.L.A. group's studies. There has been, then, in the last twenty years general agreement on the neurological basis for the deficits seen in autism, though the exact causes and mechanisms remain unclear, and probably are varied.

Meanwhile, the Skinnerian school of behaviorism had grown to dominate psychology and special education in the United States. In Skinner's view, the cause of behavior was irrelevant. If desirable behavior was rewarded and undesirable behavior unrewarded or negatively reinforced (punished), then behavior could be "shaped" into whatever pattern was desired by the person controlling rewards and punishments. The simplicity of the theory was very attractive, and the fact that almost anyone could be taught to carry it out made it a relatively inexpensive technique.

The prevailing view of neurologists was (and still appears to be) that if medication or surgery cannot be used, then there is nothing to be done to remediate the basic deficits. This lack of hope for improved nervous system function, plus the prevailing behavioristic approach in education led to a "training" paradigm whereby, it was hoped, through operant conditioning, tightly structured environments and endless repetition, the individual could be trained to respond in socially acceptable ways and to carry out at least minimal self-care activities.

Our experience in watching this philosophy in action was that it was not effective. At best it produced robots who lacked any spark of spontaneity. At worst it seemed to increase the very behaviors it was designed to eliminate. Our work at Arizona State Hospital in ferreting out sensory integrative dysfunction as a component in chronic process schizophrenia[7] led us directly to the same components in the autistic children with whom we worked. Ayres'[8,9] writings plus Ornitz' designation of autism as a sensory integrative disorder led us to try some remedial activities and the results were encouraging. The gains that were made were lasting in contrast to the results of operant conditioning which, even its proponents concede, do not carry over and do not generalize.

With the establishment at the Center of *Good Beginnings*, an intensive therapy program for 2-1/2 through 5 year olds, we began to see an occasional young autistic child. The results of 5 to 12 hours a week of therapy were, once again, encouraging to us and a source of new hope for parents. As these children approached school age, the parents faced a dilemma. The public and private school programs that were available all had the same behavioristic approach. Occupational therapy, when it was available at all, was a very minor part of the program. Children were seen in most cases only once or twice a week for forty-five minutes or less.

In 1982 we developed a curriculum according to the guidelines of the state department of education, set forth our philosophy (Figure I) and plowed through a mountain of paper work. One of our *Good Beginnings* staff was a certified special education teacher who thoroughly believed in sensory integration. In due time we were certified by the State Department of Education. We had one child of school age whose parents insisted to their school district that they wanted their son in our program. That district had serious misgivings about the *Developmental Day School*, but as the parents persisted, the school district contracted with us for that year.

The first year the *Developmental Day School* consisted of one child, one teacher, one occupational therapist. The tuition for one child obviously was not enough to support the program. Our student's mother was also a special education teacher and she offered to volunteer as a staff person in the *Good Beginnings* program in

Philosophy

The Philosophy of the Developmental Day School is that:

1. Learning depends on progressive levels of maturation of the nervous system.

2. Maturation can be facilitated through the application of neurodevelopmental principles to children's learning activities.

3. Children learn best when as many sensory and motor pathways are utilized as possible.

4. Children learn most quickly what seems to them relevant to their needs and interests.

5. Learning experiences succeed best when structured to fit each child's level of neurodevelopment, learning style, and felt needs and interests.

6. Parents should be intimately involved in understanding their child's level of maturation, setting learning goals, and following through with home activities.

In regard to multiple handicapped (autistic) children, it is the school's belief based on study of the research, that autism is a nervous system disorder and that:

1. The human brain is plastic, and there is a redundancy of neural pathways. Therefore, even in damaged or seriously delayed nervous systems, activation of alternate pathways is possible.

2. Effective teaching/learning strategies are best planned and executed by multi-disciplinary teams of educators, therapists, psychologists and parents.

3. For the handicapped child efforts should be directed toward building independent functioning in daily living skills as a foundation for maximizing the child's potential.

4. For the handicapped child, as for every other child, a paramount goal is happiness, based on a feeling of self-worth and competence fostered by the respect and love of the adults in the child's life.

To that end, the Developmental Day School will never use shaming or denigration as a method of discipline.

Self control will be fostered by structuring environment and time in positive ways.

Positive reinforcement will be used. Intrinsic motivation will be fostered by frequently verbally listing for the child what he has accomplished.

FIGURE 1

Developmental Day School

order to ease the financial burden on the Center. Since the occupational therapist (the author) was also a volunteer, the school was able to survive its first year.

The following year there were four students, the next year six, and at present, eight, which is the limit for one classroom.

Staff consists of a teacher, a full time occupational therapist, two aides, a music therapist who devotes half time to the school program, and a speech therapist who is present two mornings per week. Usually there are two occupational therapy interns in the program, as well as an occasional nursing student or music therapy student. The author is the Director of the program and is still a volunteer.

The program time is 5 hours per day, 5 days per week. Lunch is part of the program and provides opportunity for working on proper eating habits, table manners, setting and clearing the table, etc. Several of the children need improved chewing patterns and lip and tongue mobility. A period of oral motor facilitation precedes lunch for these children.

The aim of the *Developmental Day School* is to place the child in a less restrictive, i.e., more normal educational environment, as soon as he is able to benefit. Children are gradually prepared for a transition to public school by being "mainstreamed" in playground activities, in music classes, and in library periods. The location of the Center — rented space in an elementary school — makes this kind of mainstreaming possible. The Center rents five classrooms plus office space. The *Developmental Day School* occupies one classroom, the *Good Beginnings* program occupies another, and the other three rooms are therapy areas shared by both programs and used in the afternoon for individual therapy. The classrooms are also equipped with swings, trampoline, and other sensory integration equipment, so that in actuality every room is a therapy room.

The eight children in the school are divided into three groups and rotate through the classroom, an outdoor play area, and the therapy room. The classroom time focuses on a continuum of goals ranging from attending behavior to reading and filling out a job application. The special education teacher uses the child's sensory motor needs in planning the approach to academics. For example, writing or prewriting activities might be done in shaving cream on a smooth surface or by forming letters with play dough. Or a child might read while sitting on a T-stool.

A great deal of pre-academic work centers around the acquisition of basic concepts. Autistic children, who usually exhibit abnormal vestibular system function, lack position in space concepts such as up, over, between, behind, through, etc. The therapeutic activities, which tend to normalize sensory processing, also provide opportunities for learning these crucial concepts in action. These concepts are necessary for reading readiness and for following directions.

The gross motor activities of therapy which involve acquiring body concept may also assist in developing number concepts.

The outdoor time features a selection of tactile activities more suited to outdoor space, such as cornstarch and water, sandbox, or water play. Children are pulled from this area for individual sessions with the music therapist and the speech therapist.

Music is a very important modality for the autistic child since most respond very positively to it, and singing is often the beginning of oral language. In addition, the music therapist is very knowledgeable about sensory integration theory and works closely with the occupational therapist in establishing goals. For example, crossing the midline is facilitated by setting up the instruments so that the child must reach into contralateral space to play the drum or the glockenspiel. Music is combined with motor planning in rhythmic games and simple dances which also facilitate bilateral integration. The music therapist also conducts group music every morning during the universal "circle time" or "opening exercises." As one might expect, speech therapy goals are also incorporated into music time.

Spontaneous communication rather than rote "naming" is the goal of the language development program. A combination of oral and signed language is used. If oral language develops, signed words gradually drop out. For the child who cannot speak, signing becomes a very important communication tool. The child is motivated to communicate if he finds that it is a tool for manipulating his world for his pleasure. Therefore, we begin by responding immediately to the child's attempts to communicate, whether it be by words, gestures, or simply pulling the therapist over to a favorite toy. As the child finds he can elicit a response from adults, he expands his efforts. The adults, in turn, can gradually shape the child's communication into oral or manual language.

The speech pathologist-audiologist evaluates each child, and works with each child individually at least once a week and helps guide the other staff in the development of communication.

In the therapy room the occupational therapist works on specific developmental goals through "play" activities, ranging from obstacle courses to calming deep pressure activities or slow rhythmic swinging. The goals of communication and academic readiness are also incorporated into this time period. Each segment of the child's day is geared toward reinforcing all of the goals for the child.

Once a week the physical therapist is available to evaluate gait, muscle tone, and suggest remedial activities for the varied orthopedic problems which are almost universally present. These range from tight hamstrings to scoliosis to congenital absence of small muscles in the shoulder girdle. The physical therapist may watch other staff and make suggestions or may demonstrate remedial activities. Each visit is documented in the child's record. Staff frequently work together in sessions, trading the leadership or direction of the session back and forth. The close coordination of staff extends to parents who are very definitely part of the treatment team.

Individualized education plans are drawn up or revised twice a year in cooperation with parents, whose goals for their child are a prime consideration. Communication with parents often occurs daily since some parents transport their students. For the others, a weekly telephone call is the rule and may be supplemented as needed. Suggestions for home activities are provided and every effort is made to have behavior management strategies consistent between home and school. In addition, parents are encouraged to avail themselves of the information in the progress notes at frequent intervals and are free to come in and read their child's chart at any time. Staff are very much aware that having a child for 5 hours a day, 5 days a week is far different from having them 24 hours a day. We believe it is important for parents to meet the needs of their non-handicapped children, as well as those of the autistic child. We should not add to parents' burdens by having unreasonable expectations as to what they can do at home.

A major difference between the *Developmental Day School* and other schools for autistic children is the way in which self-stimulating or self-abusive behaviors are handled. In the first place these behaviors are related to stress. They are engaged in because they are calming to the child. Therefore, these behaviors can provide a cue to staff to remove stressors or remove the child from the stressful situation. Noise is the most common stressor. Too many people coming and going around the child is the second most common stressor which may be related to tactile defensiveness. Demands the child does not understand or cannot meet are also common stressors.

Secondly, the nature of the self-stimulating behavior is regarded as a clue as to what sensory modality is most needed by the child for organizing his sensory inputs and motor responses. As socially acceptable means for meeting these needs are provided, the unacceptable patterns drop out. For example, the child who rocks responds to swinging. At first, he or she may swing for long periods of time, but this need gradually diminishes and the rocking also diminishes and eventually disappears, except under extreme stress.

This method of handling self-stimulating or self-abusive behaviors is much more effective than operant conditioning which does not generalize from one setting to another and does not have a lasting effect. Also, "negative reinforcement" of self-stimulating or self-abusive behaviors often increases the stress the child experiences and may actually increase the behavior it is designed to eliminate.

The *Developmental Day School* is too new to have accumulated a great deal of outcome data. However, one child has graduated to a language disorder program and another is soon to graduate to a learning disability classroom in a public school.

The *Developmental Day School* is gradually winning acceptance by school districts. As directors of special education visit the program, they note that there is little self stimulating behavior and that the children are happy and smiling. In addition the records show significant improvements in scores on various achievement tests. Parents are pleased with results.

The Center's goal in establishing the *Developmental Day School* is to provide a model or a demonstration school which may serve to motivate others to try similar methods. The temptation to expand into a large program will be resisted and it is planned that the school will never exceed three classrooms serving primary, intermediate and adolescent groups.

To date the project is professionally rewarding, though it remains financially tenuous. It is hoped that grant support for research, which is in its beginning stages, will be forthcoming. Research data to support the positive results for which there is currently experiential validation will be important in encouraging others to adopt a sensory-integrative-neurodevelopmental approach.

REFERENCES

1. Kanner, L: Autistic disturbances of affective contact. *Nerv Child* 2217-250, 1943

2. Ornitz, EM: Childhood Autism: A disorder of sensorimotor integration. *Int'l Rev of Research in Ment Retard* 1(3), 50-68, 1970

3. Rimland, B: *Infantile Autism: The Syndrome and its Implications for a Neural Theory of Behavior*. New York: Appleton Century-Crofts Inc., 1964

4. Wing L, Wing JK: Multiple impairments in early childhood autism. *J Autism Child Schizo* 1: 256-266, 1971

5. Bender, L: Schizophrenia in childhood. *Am J Orthopsychiatry* 26: 499-550, 1956

6. Fish, B, Hagin, R: Visual-motor disorders in infants at risk for schizophrenia. *Arch of Gen Psychiat* 27: 594-598, 1972

7. King, LD: A sensory-integrative approach to schizophrenia *Am J Occ Ther* 28: 529-536, 1978

8. Ayres, AJ: *Sensory Integration and Learning Disorders*, Los Angeles, Calif: Western Psychological Services, 1972

9. Ayres, AJ: Sensory integrative dysfunction in Autism. *Proceedings of Seventh Annual Conference of the National Society for Autistic Children*. New York: National Society for Autistic Children, pp. 4-9, 1975

Sensory Integration
and Ego Development
in a Schizophrenic Adolescent Male

Karen A. Pettit, MEd, OTR/L

SUMMARY. This single case study of a schizophrenic adolescent presents a detailed analysis of gains in ego functions and clinical observations. A time out record was retrospectively compiled. The purpose of the time out record was to evaluate the generalized effects of sensory integrative treatment procedures on the client's ability to deal with anger and frustration in his living environment. Statistical analysis did not yield a significant difference between pre- and post-treatment data. The results of this study demonstrate the usefulness of statistical analysis verses visual comparison of pre- and post-treatment data in the validation of treatment effectiveness. Visual inspection might support a conclusion of a significant difference, when statistic analysis will not.

Although marked decreases were noted in the client's time out record as he mastered hypersensitivity to movement, development of protective extension, and gravitational security no direct statistical link could be made to the sensory integration treatment intervention. This case study does however, lay a foundation for relating ego development to vestibular system function.

Our job as occupational therapists is to utilize the patients' healthy areas of strength and nurture or maximize their normal

---

Karen A. Pettit is an assistant professor in Occupational Therapy at the University of New England. At the time of this study, she was the assistant director of the Occupational Therapy Department at Warren State Hospital, Warren, PA. Inquiries about this article may be sent to the author at UNE, College of Arts and Sciences, 11 Hills Beach Road, Biddeford, ME 04005.

Acknowledgement: The author would like to acknowledge Joe for his helping me to understand and appreciate the value of a clinician's trust in the client to promote growth. His never-ending patience and acceptance of me has been one of my most prized gifts as a therapist.

This article appears jointly in *Sensory Integrative Approaches in Occupational Therapy* (The Haworth Press, 1987) and *Occupational Therapy in Health Care*, Volume 4, Number 2 (Summer 1987).

functioning without immobilizing them with fear and tension. It is dignity, the freedom to explore, and trust that will help the patients to establish or re-establish faith and hope in their own abilities.

Ayres[1,p.128] states "the 'urge to live' should be tapped, for it is the greatest source of motivation that leads to adaptive responses and without it the therapist is relatively helpless."

In order for growth to occur, one's innate drive to survive must be nurtured with successful and challenging tasks. The continuum of complexity, quality and effectiveness of response is the life long process of adaptation.

THEORETICAL LINK
BETWEEN EGO DEVELOPMENT
AND THE VESTIBULAR SYSTEM

Menninger[2] describes the ego as the apparatus that perceives, decides, and regulates how to deal with incoming stimuli, instinctual urges, and reality in order to maintain a steady state of equilibrium and homeostasis. It is the ego that must have an external orientation. It must be perceptually sensitive and discriminating in an internal direction to permit constructive shifts in the level of homeostasis to allow growth, development and the realization of potentialities.

Menninger[2] considers the ego as the controlling mechanism which recognizes, receives, stores, discriminates, integrates and acts by restraining, releasing, modifying and directing the impulses. Frick[3] describes Hartmann's concept of ego as an integrator and organizer within the personality. One's physical, cognitive and emotional self perceptions are organized by the ego. The ego balances, integrates and stabilizes the libidinal and aggressive drives. The maintenance of one's self identity is an integrative function of the ego. If one agrees with both Menninger and Hartmann then the question is raised as to what influences the ego in order to promote higher level adaptive responses for our patients. Could the neurological counterpart of ego mechanisms be partially or wholly accounted for by the vestibular, reticular and the limbic system functioning? For the purposes of this paper the role of the vestibulocerebellar system in ego development will be addressed.

The labyrinths are the specific portions of the vestibulocerebellar system that are sensitive to acceleration and deceleration of motion.

They are the structures that are responsible for the body's orientation and internal sense of direction. The otoliths of the utricule sand accule are concerned with position and gravity perception. Schilder[4] states that dizziness is a sign that the ego is in danger because it cannot exercise its synthetic function in the senses, or because conflicting motor and attitudinal impulses in relation to desires and strivings can no longer be united. Changes in the vestibulocerebellar system's role of organizing and integrating of information may be reflected in psyche structures, one of which is the ego. Murphy[5] in her work with children describes two levels of coping. The first and most basic coping patterns that must be established are the ones that deal with the opportunities, frustrations and obstacles within the physical environment. The second level of coping is the maintenance of internal equilibrium, the one's ability to deal with his temperament and people within his environment. If one's reflexes, and sensory motor development are poorly integrated then coping becomes much more difficult. The second level of coping is much harder to achieve. Feldenkrais[6] states the infant's first unconditional fear is gravity or falling and that the infant must establish a trust relationship with the environment.

It would then seem that the two vestibulocerebellar functions that must be mastered in order to successfully adapt and cope with people are: (a) to establish a trust and mastery of the fear of falling and, (b) to establish a maintenance of internal equilibrium through a stable visual field. These two functions permit successful orientation to one's physical environment prior to establishing a trust relationship with people.

White[7] suggests that the adaptive process and coping process involve the simultaneous management of securing adequate information, maintaining satisfactory internal conditions, and keeping a degree of autonomy. The author suggests that the vestibulocerebellar system may have a pervasive and powerful effect on the organization and gathering of information necessary for the ego development.

CASE STUDY

A single case study will demonstrate the effectiveness of occupational therapy intervention while using sensory integrative techniques in the area of ego development.

Description of the Subject

Joe was referred to occupational therapy by a physician after being identified as demonstrating right-left hesitancy problems (difficulties with right-left discrimination) on neurological examination, destructive, aggressive, and immature social behaviors that persisted 2 years after his admission to the adolescent unit in a large state institution.

Joe was thirteen at the time of his admission to the adolescent unit. At the age of three he was taken from his mother as a result of gross neglect and abuse; he had been placed in three foster homes and hospitalized for cruelty to animals. He was admitted to the adolescent unit from a children's home because of auditory and visual hallucinations, feelings of sadness, and difficulty with word-finding during speech. His history included stealing and fire setting. His intelligence scores varied from 55 to 80. At the time of his admission his chief complaint was "I want help with listening and seeing." His behavior on the unit included hyperactivity, destructiveness, verbal and physical threats, and he related to others through kicking, hitting and temper tantrums. He was defiant, assaultive, and destroyed property with acts such as setting fires, flooding bathrooms, ripping plaster from walls, and disassembling iron beds, heating register grates and protective heater cages.

Joe was 15 years and 3 months old at the time he was referred to occupational therapy. He was diagnosed as Schizophrenic, Childhood Type with Borderline Mental Retardation. The Southern California Sensory Integration Tests (SCSIT) were administered to evaluate his ability to organize and utilize sensory input before and after treatment. Since his age was beyond the limit of the normative data for the tests, raw scores in addition to clinical observations were used for evaluation.

Evaluation Results

The results of the evaluation suggested that Joe had developmental dyspraxia that seemed to stem from a related vestibular processing disorder evidenced by poor prone extension, poor balance, low muscle tone, poor equilibrium, and problems with gravitational insecurity, tactile defensiveness, and distractibility. End products of poor eye-hand coordination (design copying, bilateral coordination and lack of a skilled dominant hand) were some of his functional problems evident from the testing. Areas of deficit ego development that were critical to Joe's adjustment in everyday living were his difficulties communicating anger and frustration, lack of age appropriate play and social relationships, poor impulse control and poor judgement.

Treatment Program

Treatment sessions consisted of three two hour sessions of occupational therapy per week for one year. Joe was treated in a group of six to ten adolescents. He received at least one half hour of individualized occupational therapy utilizing a sensory integrative approach each session while two other staff members implemented group activities designed to facilitate age appropriate play and social responses. During Joe's sensory integrative treatment time others in the group received sedentary arts and crafts and noncompetitive gross motor activities, running, exercises, hiking, and musical activities. Much of Joe's first 3 months in sensory integrative treatment was spent exploring activities with his head in an inverted position, and neck and shoulder joint compression activities. As Joe's ability to process vestibular input improved, sensory integrative treatment sessions included linear accelerated movement while prone on the scooter board, vertical linear movement on a make shift trampoline and then a gradually expanded repertoire of activities to include rotary and linear vestibular input using suspended platform swings and hammocks. As his equilibrium reactions improved, and his processing of antigravity positions became comfortable, activities such as rolling with the support of touch pressure, linear movement while supine in a hammock, and climbing activities were initiated.

DOCUMENTATION OF TREATMENT EFFECTIVENESS

In order to measure the effectiveness of the sensory integration techniques in occupational therapy, a retrospective study was done to compare the number of hours Joe spent in "time out" each month prior to the initiation of occupational therapy to the hours he spent in "time out" while he was receiving treatment. The purpose of the time out measure was to evaluate the improvements noted in both vestibular system processing and ego development gains in such a way that generalizations could be seen back on his unit. Table 1 compares Joe's "time out" record for both the baseline year and the treatment year.

Joe's "time out" baseline was analyzed utilizing the "C" statistic process, Ottenbacher,[8] to determine whether a significant change occurred. Essentially the baseline data is analyzed to determine if it contains a significant existing trend. If there is no significant trend, then the baseline data and treatment data can be combined and analyzed to determine the existence of a significant difference across both the baseline and intervention phases.

When Joe's baseline data was analyzed with the "C" statistic, a score of 4.132 was obtained. This result demonstrated a high level of significance, indicative of an existing decline in "time out" in the baseline, pretreatment phase. Therefore, the intervention phase could not be compared with the baseline phase to determine the effects of the intervention.

Joe's "time out" data during the intervention phase had the same slope as the baseline above and below the celeration line. This indicates that no significant difference was seen in the effectiveness of the intervention. The decline in Joe's "time out" record during treatment could not be statistically linked to the intervention due to the apparent prexisting deceleration of his time spent in "time out."

TABLE 1

HOURS IN TIME OUT

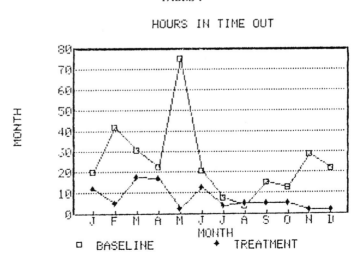

□   BASELINE   ✦   TREATMENT

One should note that during the months of July and August the pre-treatment time out was zero. During these months Joe was in bilateral casts after foot surgery.

To document improvement in ego development, behaviors reflecting the twelve ego functions as outlined by Bellak et al.[9] were recorded. Appendix A lists examples of Joe's behaviors in each ego function prior to and after one year of treatment. Table 2 displays the changes in Joe's ego development between the two years. Changes noted in Joe's ego development during treatment were dramatic in many areas. He was able to cooperatively play, and ask for assistance when becoming upset. He progressed from physical abuse of others to primarily verbal abuse of others. Engagement in group activities without incident and a move from severe narcissistic and sadistic tendencies to becoming somewhat sensitive to others potential rejection were hallmarks in his social interactions. He began to make connections between his actions and other's reactions. Reduced sensory thresholds occurred during stressful situations which enabled him to engage in more age appropriate activities. His mastery of gravitational insecurity, hypersensitivity to movement and tactile defensiveness enabled him to concentrate more directly on interpersonal interactions when engaged in activities.

CONCLUSIONS

There are several implications of this case study. There was no significant statistical evidence of the effectiveness of the occupational therapy intervention as measured by the "time out" record. However the changes Joe made in the area of ego function were striking and supported by the tendency of decline in his "time out" record as he made improvements in processing vestibular information. Vestibular processing gains were seen as decreased hypersensitivity to rotary movement as well as evidence of the development of the protective extension response and gains in gravitational security. The major improvement in behavior was Joe's attempts to cooperatively play and initiate a broader range of activities during treatment. Simultaneously with his gains in the vestibular system his "time out" record decreased and steadily dropped as further gains were made in motor performance. Although this cannot be attributed to occupational therapy alone due to the baseline tendency in this direction, the author feels that the vestibular input as a

TABLE 2

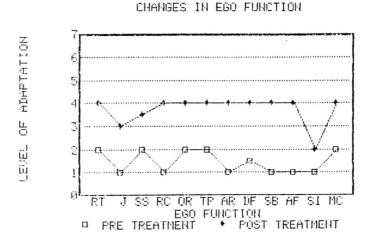

CHANGES IN EGO FUNCTION

□ PRE TREATMENT   ✦ POST TREATMENT

part of occupational therapy intervention was a vital component of change. Marked improvements in ego changes were noted: Joe's ability to control his affect and impulses, adaptive regression in the service of his ego, awareness of stimulus barriers, improved autonomous functioning and in his uses of defensive functioning.

This case suggests that perhaps goals of occupational therapy using a sensory integrative model could be to reduce the stress on the ego in order for the individual to master and develop his adaptive capacity within the environment. This is done through helping the patient organize a successful adaptation to movement and gravity through the normalization of the vestibular system. The treatment media are purposeful activities involving vestibular, proprioceptive, and tactile input. The second goal of treatment might focus on helping the patient discover the stimulation he needs to maintain his optimum level of adaptation. This can be done through maintained amounts of stimulation, movement and activity. Through the vestibular system treatment activities it would appear one's ability to cope can be raised from a successful adaptation of the physical environment to one of internal maintenance and equilibrium. The primitive ego coping mechanisms described by Menninger[3] seeking touch, vestibular input to calm, and limbic system releases like laughter, crying, swearing, and sleeping could then be augmented with the development of higher level coping mechanisms. Such things as the enhancement of communication through occupational therapy using sensory integrative techniques which enable one to better express conflicts and frustrations, or through working off excess energy/aggression through the muscular system could be used. Both mechanisms, the enhancement of communication and successful participation in age appropriate activities due to mastery of environmental adaptations are potential end products of ego development that has been facilitated in this adolescent using a sensory integrative model of treatment.

REFERENCES

1. Ayres AJ: *Sensory Integration and Learning Disorders*. Los Angeles, CA: Western Psychological Services, 1972, p. 128

2. Menninger KA: Psychological Aspects of the Organism Under Stress. *J Amer Psychoanalytic Assoc* 2: 67-106, 1954

3. Frick RB: The Ego and the Vestibulocerebellar System: Some Theoretical Perspectives. *Psychoanalytic Quarterly* 14: 93-122, 1982

4. Schilder, P: The Vestibular Apparatus in Neurosis and Psychosis. *J Nerv & Ment Dis* 78: 1-164, 1933

5. Murphy LB: Coping, Vulnerability, and Resilience in Childhood. In *Coping and Adaptation*, GV Coelho, Editor. New York: Basic Books, 69-100, 1974

6. Feldenkrais M: *Body & Mature Behavior*. New York, NY: International Univ Press, 1979

7. White RW: Strategies of Adaptation: An Attempt at Systematic Description. In *Coping and Adaptation*, GV Coelho, Editor. New York: Basic Books, 47-68, 1974

8. Ottenbacher KJ: *Evaluating Clinical Change*. Baltimore, MD: Williams & Wilkins, 1986

9. Bellak L, Hurvich M, Gediman H: *Ego Functions in Schizophrenics, Neurotics, and Normals*. New York, NY: John Wiley & Sons, 1973

APPENDIX A

JOE'S EGO DEVELOPMENT DURING ONE YEAR OF OCCUPATIONAL THERAPY
USING A SENSORY INTEGRATIVE MODEL
(The higher the number the more adaptive the behavior on a scale from 1-7).

*EGO FUNCTION	*EGO COMPONENT DEFINED	JOE'S BEHAVIORS
REALITY TESTING (RT)	Separation between internal/external stimuli.	Pre Rx: (2) Did not realize he fantasized. Believed he was the Incredible Hulk and Superman.
		Post Rx: (4) Progressed to projection of inner states, acknowledged awareness that fantasy was not real. Desired to have me show that he was important through total attention. He projected this through Doctor/Nurse fantasy play.
	Accurate perception of external (time/place) and internal events.	Pre Rx: (1) Inability to provide reasons to explain behavior and feelings. Little awareness of when he felt sad, angry, happy or loving. For no apparent reason, Joe would become angry and throw a chair at a peer.
		Post Rx: (4) Moderate degree of awareness from within self. Could play cooperatively with another peer, ask for the object he wanted, could verbalize that he needed and wanted assistance, was aware when he began to get upset.
JUDGEMENT (J)	Anticipation of consequences. (legal, social, physical harm)	Pre Rx: (1) Verbal and physical aggression. Fire setting and theft. Separated from parents for abuse of animals, people and fire setting.
		Post Rx: (3) Anticipated "time out" for destructive behaviors. No longer setting fires and throwing chairs/furniture. Mostly verbal abuse towards others.
	Behavior reflects awareness of likely consequences. (repetition of behaviors)	Pre Rx: (1) Numerous foster home/ institutional placements since age of three. Spent 304 hours in "time out" the year prior to OT treatment.
		Post Rx: (3) 97 hours in "time out" during one year of OT treatment.
	Appropriateness of behavior to external social/ emotional/physical situations	Pre Rx: (1) Throws furniture when frustrated/angry. Disassembles furniture, floods bathrooms. Initiates fights with others when attention is not solely on him.
		Post Rx: (3) Increased social awareness and value placed on peer interactions. Required help identifying options when in conflict.

*Bellak L., Hurvich M, Gediman,H: *Ego Functions In Schizophrenics, Neurotics, and Normals*: Wiley and Sons New York, 1973

APPENDIX A (continued)

SENSE OF REALITY OF THE WORLD AND OF THE SELF (SS)	Experience of external events as real.	
	Feeling of one's body parts and functions as belonging to oneself.	
	Degree of development of individuality, uniqueness an a sense of self and self esteem.	Pre Rx: (2) Self esteem is poor. Much make-believe about trying to be boss.
	Degree of separation of one's self from objects.	Pre Rx: (2) When feedback from others is not there, his sense of self falters.
		Post Rx: (3.5) Able to provide positive feedback to others in group.
REGULATION AND CONTROL OF DRIVE, AFFECT AND IMPULSE (RC)	Directness of impulse expression.	Pre Rx: (1) Physical expression of anger and frustration. Sets fires and physical abuse to both animals and people. Did not regulate any primitive feelings.
		Post Rx: (4) Able to share; able to
	Effectiveness of delayed mechanisms	take turns on equipment and toys. Able to engage in group activity without incident.
OBJECT RELATIONS (OR)	The degree and kind of relatedness to others.	Pre Rx: (2) Severe narcissistic, sadomasochistic relationships. Derives pleasure from exercising power over others. Hit and teased
	The extent to which present relationships are patterned upon or influenced by older ones and serve present mature aims rather than past immature ones.	until he made others cry or until they did what he wanted. No recognition of other's feelings or motives. Verbally and physically expressed anger of loss of record player and cape he used in his fantansy. Sharing or change in activity caused catastrophic results.
	Object constancy, the sustaining of physical absence of the object and the present mature aims rather than past immature ones.	Post Rx: (4) Sensitive to others potential rejections. Cooperative play and interaction. Attempts to get others to change rather than to accept them. Relationships are characterized by game playing and Don Juanism.
THOUGHT PROCESSES (TP)	Adequacy of processes that guide and sustain thought (attention, concentration, anticipation, concept formation, memory and language.	Pre Rx: (2) Attention and concentration is poor. Easily distracted by visual & auditory stimuli. Requires 1:1 attention in order to complete any simple craft or ADL task. Illogical sequence in his communication. Frequently blocks when trying to describe events or interactions. Difficulty seeing connections between what he does and consequences of his behavior.

APPENDIX A (continued)

The extent to which thinking is unrealistic, illogical and/or loose. (primary/secondary thinking.

Post Rx: (4) Makes connections between his actions and reactions. Realizes that teasing keeps others distant or makes them tease him. Able to complete activities with 2 step directions independently. Attends to a task approximately 20-30 minutes without distraction from others in the group. Gives eye contact and wants to make sure he has your total attention before he speaks.

ARISE
Adaptive
Regression in
Service of the
Ego

(AR)

Regressive relaxation perceptual & cognitive acuity.

Pre Rx: (1) Regressions are primitive and prominant. He hits, kicks or throws when he perceives a threat. A threat to him is someone else who gets attention, accomplishes an activity, comes too close to him (4-10 feet), or has something he wants to do. Viewed things as throwing or kicking objects. Unable to generalize now to constructively play with toys.

Extent of increased adaptive potential expressed in new configurations and creative integrations.

Post Rx: (4) He discovered how to utilize several toys to create fantansies to help him cope with the pressures from other group members. He initiated bringing others into his play because it made the fantasy more fun. Tended not to easily shift fantasy play into skill development or serious discussion.

DEFENSIVE
FUNCTIONING
(DF)

Extent to which defense mechanisms affected ideation, behavior, and the adaptive level.

Pre Rx: (1.5) Pervasive feeling of vulnerability. Majority of interactions perceived as attacks or threats to personal worth. Constant use of denial and projection. Emergence of id desires. Pathologic identification with any aggressor. Free-floating anxiety.

Extent to which defenses have succeeded or failed. Degree of anxiety, depression, dysphoric affects.

Post Rx: (4) Evidence of rationalization and reaction-formation. Fantasy is a substitute for repressed thoughts. States he is the strongest man in the world when attempting to deal with the anxiety of how to cope with older men on his unit. When he can't find solutions, he reverts back to primitive, immature behaviors but ones that are somewhat less harmful. i.e. throwing match books down vents rather than setting fires, verbal threats instead of physical ones, fantasies of power rather than bombs and destruction.

STIMULUS
BARRIER
(SB)

Threshold for sensitivity to, or registration of external and internal experiences which impinge upon function.

Pre Rx: (1) Hypersensitive to movement, head or body orientation, visual/tactile stimuli, and sounds. Control of frustration and anger at himself due to lack of control over environmental stimuli i.e. unable to engage in activities like gymnastics wrestling, and swimming because he gets dizzy and sick when he has

APPENDIX A (continued)

to roll or rotate his body. Fears a loss of control when swimming if his feet don't touch the ground. Perceives any spontaneous touch as threat or attacks. He becomes destructive to avoid the reality of not being successful in those activities.

The effectiveness of coping mechanism in relation to degree of sensory stimulation (motor, affective and cognitive)

Post Rx: (4) Reduced sensory thresholds occur under stressed situations. Able to engage in swimming, wrestling and competitive running relays. Able to engage in conversations without distractions of movements and sounds. Able to entertain self for 20-30 minutes.

AUTONOMUS FUNCTIONING (AF)

Degree of freedom from impairment of primary autonomy (sight, hearing, intention, language, memory, learning, motor function, intelligence)

Pre Rx: (1) Efforts at willful performances are virtually ineffective. Inability to concentrate or attend no matter how much effort is invested. Unable to learn without 1:1 instruction in distraction free environment. No well established interests, daily habits or basic work skills.

Degree of freedom from impairment of secondary autonomy (habit patterns, complex learned skills, work routines, interests and hobbies)

Post Rx: (4) Aggressive thoughts and fantasies interfer with his finding appropriate words, and in performing motor behaviors. Joe would get so upset he would trip and stutter and lose his concentration. If a new assignment came at work or if new staff member came onto the unit, he would be unable to keep himself organized.

SYNTHETIC-INTEGRATIVE FUNCTIONING (SI)

Degree of reconciliation or integration of contradictory attitudes, values, affects, behaviors, & self-representations.

Pre Rx: (1) Minimal ability to have congruent affect i.e: laughing while throwing a chair at a peer in the group.. Cannot cope with more than one task at a time. Unable to implement an activity according to a plan.

Degree of integration of psychic & behavioral events.

Post Rx: (2) Organized treatment session by determining equipment he wanted to use and then would interact constructively with the environment. Developed feelings of remorse and identified that aggressive outbursts could be harmful to others.

MASTERY-COMPETENCE (MC)

Degree of difference between actual competence and sense of competence.

Pre Rx: (2) Higher than actual competence. Confuses what he'd like to be able to do with what he can do. Controls all actions of others. Successful interactions with the environment come from manipulation of people or waiting for things to happen. Can protect himself against peer teasing and authority thru physical force and threats. Does not problem solve. Can not control his response to environment; wants only to control the people in it.

The person's feeling of competence with mastering and affecting his environment.

APPENDIX A (continued)

How well the person actually performs in relation to his existing capacity to interact act & master his environment.

Post Rx: (4) Mastered control of his response to movement, gravitational insecurity and tactile defensiveness which enabled him to focus more directly on interpersonal relationships and skill development.

A Sensory Integration Based Program with a Severely Retarded/Autistic Teenager: An Occupational Therapy Case Report

Geraldene G. Larrington, MA, OTR

SUMMARY. This case report illustrates occupational therapy based on sensory integration philosophy and treatment principles with a severely mentally retarded/autistic fifteen year old boy. Evaluation, treatment and results are outlined and discussed retrospectively. An oral stimulation and feeding program is presented as an additional and integral part of his occupational therapy program. The integration of his occupational therapy program into his daily group home and school life is presented and the contribution of these other caregivers assessed.

This retrospective case report illustrates occupational therapy with a severely mentally retarded/autistic fifteen year old boy, referred to here as D. Sensory integration (SI) theory, philosophy and

Mrs. Larrington is currently Occupational Therapist at the Arizona School for the Deaf and Blind in Tucson, AZ.

Acknowledgements: The author extends special thanks to Lorna Jean King, OTR; Paula Weisbrodt-Kelly, MS, OTR; Marsha Dunn, MEd, OTR; Dona DeClusin, OTR; David Sibbles (and school aides); George Franklin (and group home staff); and D's family.

This paper was adapted from a presentation at the 1986 Second Annual Autism Conference in Tucson, Arizona, sponsored by the Pima County Chapter of the National Society for Children and Adults with Autism.

This article appears jointly in *Sensory Integrative Approaches in Occupational Therapy* (The Haworth Press, 1987) and *Occupational Therapy in Health Care*, Volume 4, Number 2 (Summer 1987).

treatment principles were the basis for D's initial occupational therapy treatment program. As needs were identified and as his behavior, attention span and ability to cooperate improved, his program was complemented and augmented by the addition of other occupational therapy skills such as oral sensory-motor stimulation, neuromuscular facilitation and neurodevelopmental techniques. Sensory integration theory and philosophy, however, continued to guide D's therapy intervention.

BACKGROUND

D's primary diagnosis has always been severe mental retardation with the autistic behaviors identified secondarily. Chromosomal studies were normal and no definitive neurological assessment has suggested possible sites of dysfunction.

D is small for his age but his health has been generally good. Hearing and vision have been considered medically normal and functional. Although he has no speech, his receptive language has always been a strength and he has acquired some sign language. He presented a flexion pattern in his standing and walking postures along with a wide-based stance.

His intelligence quotient (IQ) has been estimated to be between 19 and 32, with a Vineland Social Maturity Scale Social Age of 3 years 5 months. His educational placement has been in a Trainable Mentally Retarded/Multiply Handicapped class with consultation from occupational therapy, physical therapy, adaptive physical education and speech/language departments.

Concerns

D has had numerous, long-standing behaviors which were considered abusive to self and others or were otherwise destructive or problematic. These include grabbing objects, breaking and/or throwing them, plate and food throwing, bowel and bladder accidents, and pulling the hair of others as well as himself. Screeching, biting and hitting himself, biting holes in his shirts, drooling, twisting his arms up in his clothes and around his neck, leg wrapping, head banging and head snapping were also typical behaviors.

The family was increasingly concerned about D's future as well as their own in relationship to him. On visits to his group home, they could no longer physically control D to protect him, themselves, or the environment from his impulsive, seemingly destructive behaviors. They were greatly distressed that as they yearned to integrate him more fully into their lives, it was increasingly difficult to be around him. They came away mentally, emotionally and physically abused and exhausted. Moreover, they feared that he would not receive the care he needed in the future unless his behavior could be altered so that people would not become burned out, shun him or give him less love, care and attention.

This was not a new concern for the family. They had previously pursued intensive efforts to alter behavior through behavior modification techniques. These programs, as well as the traditional delivery of educational and therapy services, had yielded some slow, steady or temporary gains but not the needed major changes.

EVALUATION

Lorna Jean King, OTR, provided the initial evaluation in May, 1984, and has been able to periodically consult and make recommendations throughout treatment. Since standardized tests are not usable with such an involved child, she relied upon her extensive experience with children with similar problems, and upon observation and reports of D's behavior. She also offered him a variety of sensory experiences in order to assess his reactions to them. For example, D explored vibratory sensation with a hand-held vibrator and electric detangler; he was gently swung side to side in a net hammock by two therapists and pulled around over carpeting in the hammock; furry rug material was wrapped around his legs. She also observed drooling, poor mouth closure, as well a poor chewing and swallowing patterns during a snack of crackers.

D was found to be responsive to a variety of sensory input and could be both stimulated and calmed. His need for vibratory input was inferred from his great fascination and exploration of vibratory sources. Proprioceptive needs were inferred from his constant self-hugging through leg and arm wrapping. The need for calming activities was apparent in his general distractible and disruptive behavior. The need for an oral sensory-motor program was also established in the initial evaluation.

TREATMENT

At the Group Home

Treatment was begun in July, 1984 at the group home on a twice a week basis although it had to be reduced to once a week when school started. Treatment sessions were 45 to 60 minutes in duration. Paula Weisbrodt-Kelly, MS, OTR, a private practice occupational therapist, provided most of his therapy program.

The author was also involved in planning and directing the course of D's treatment and provided some direct therapy services as needed to relieve the primary therapist. The author interfaced with the family and school as well as the group home and handled most of the communication about the case in progress notes, summaries and letters.

In order to provide more optimal frequent therapy and also hold down the costs of private therapy, group home staff and the mother were involved in the treatment sessions and were trained to provide sensory stimulation opportunities for thirty minutes six days a week. A notebook to chart and briefly describe the activities provided was set up and used as a communication tool between the treating therapists, mother and the group home staff.

The group home staff were very responsive to the program, seemed to enjoy working with D and had no difficulty understanding how to follow D's lead regarding what type of input he sought on a particular day. The more relaxed, free-flowing atmosphere of the group home was very compatible with an occupational therapy program with its emphasis on playful, patient-directed sensory integrative activities.

A hanging net, rebounder (mini exercise trampoline), scooterboard, vibrator, weighted vest and various sources of tactile input were the earliest equipment provided. Another type of vibrator, a vibrating table and a weighted lap robe were added later. A platform swing, big ball and manipulative toys became more important in later stages of treatment.

D soon settled in on vibration as a primary input. Curled up on the rebounder as close to someone as he could get, he held the vibrator primarily on his right ear. He became very calm and relaxed for relatively long periods of time. He was encouraged to apply the vibrator elsewhere on his body, but his preference was his ear.

To calm behavior and increase postural extension, a weighted vest was worn daily for off and on periods of 20 to 60 minutes. The duration was left up to the discretion of the group home personnel based on what seemed to work best for D in the particular situation.

School Support

A consultation with the school teacher and school occupational therapist was held in the fall, resulting in the teacher incorporating more sensory integration concepts into D's daily therapy and education programs. For example, a cloth covered lead X-ray apron was placed across his lap when seated to provide proprioceptive feedback and free up his hands for signing as a substitute for his need to hug a lap table tightly into his body. Also the vibrator was made available to D for unrestricted use during free play times instead of being briefly offered as a reward for performance as it was formerly used. The school staff also cooperated with the use of the weighted vest.

Direct occupational therapy services in the school was requested and begun by Dona DeClusin, OTR, on a once-a-week basis for 30-40 minutes in December, 1984. Since the school could not provide more frequent therapy, private therapy was continued weekly to assure that D was receiving direct therapy treatment twice a week. Periodic consultation helped coordinate these therapy efforts with good results. Classroom and home programming also continued.

Oral-Motor Program Addition

In March, 1985, (eight months after the onset of the therapeutic program) a consultation from an occupational therapy specialist in oral-feeding problems with infants and young children was requested to develop the oral-motor stimulation aspects of D's occupational therapy treatment program. Marsha Dunn, MEd, OTR, was able to train the group home staff in an oral-facial stimulation and feeding program designed to decrease drooling, develop lip and mouth closure, encourage tongue lateralization of food and improve sucking, chewing and swallowing. Highlights of this oral program are described in Appendix A.

RESULTS

Numerous changes were noted throughout the course of treatment and are listed briefly in Table 1. Changes were noted subjectively in a variety of areas: physical posture, decreased problem behaviors, alertness, increased attention span and ability to cooperate, and a wider range of play, work and manipulative skills. In retrospect, an attempt has been made to document more objectively some of these changes. Both subjective and objective reports are included below.

Physical Posture

The physical changes in posture were apparent early in treatment. A more erect, extended posture with a narrower stance base also

Table 1. Summary of D's changes.

Increased/Improved:

            calmness, ability to attend and cooperate
            alertness to people and activities
            oral-motor functions: mouth closure,
                lateralized chewing, swallowing
            standing posture: less flexion
            sitting posture: upright
            self-control
            manipulative skills
            wider range of interests
            completes task or play sequence
            more functional, purposeful activities

Decreased:

            abusive, destructive acts
            head banging and snapping
            screeching
            bowel and bladder movements in pants
            biting self and shirt
            twisting arms in clothing and leg wrapping

developed. Photographs in Figure 1 illustrate change in self-selected chair sitting posture. Note the continued need to wrap the feet around chair legs. He has abandoned the W-sitting which characterized his floor sitting behavior and now spontaneously tailor sits or long sits with knees partially flexed.

In the Group Home

In the group home, meal-times and bed-times were increasingly more relaxed and life around D was more comfortable. A behavior sample probe was taken by the group home, for their own purposes, in September of 1984 (two months after therapy was begun) and another in May of 1985 (eight months later). Unfortunately the sampling techniques were not the same and therefore were not directly comparable. However, with some mathematical manipulations involving multiplying to equalize observation times and controlling for the number of days observed, the data was better reconciled and showed striking decreases in the behaviors under observation which were: head to object, head to knee, wrist to head, plate throwing and hair pulling. Because of the mathematical manipulations these are not reported here.

However, the group home did repeat the May procedure precisely in September, 1985 (4 months later). From May to September, 1985, there was a better than 50% reduction in all behaviors under observation, in addition to the earlier major reductions.

At School

Meal times at school also became more pleasant. Food and plate throwing were markedly reduced by April, 1985. The frenetic pace of his eating was tempered. For example, he could now bite a sandwich, set it down, chew and then swallow before picking it up again.

Bowel and bladder accidents were almost non-existent by the end of the term. The teacher and aides were also having to find new activities for him as his interest in his environment and responsiveness to it increased. Their time was no longer absorbed with management programs trying to get him upright, attentive, and with arms and hands free to work. He would now engage more constructively in activities such as sorting three objects (knives, forks, spoons) and identifying five basic colors on four of five trials. D

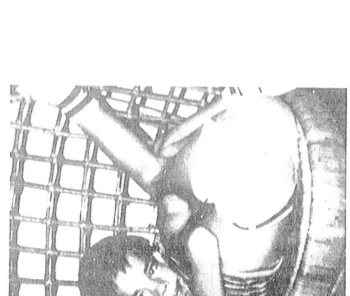

BEFORE

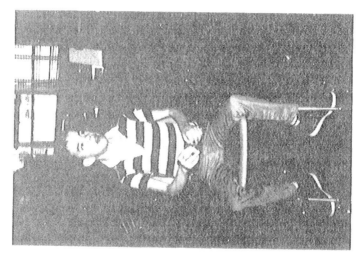

AFTER

FIGURE 1. Samples of D's Sitting Postures Before and After Treatment

could attend more calmly, with less screaming or other signs of frustration.

During the 1985-86 school year D began showing more interest in his environment and in people. For example, he chose to ride a stationary exercise bicycle instead of perseverating on old, familiar toys during free time. He also became more aware of fellow class-mates — watching them and laughing at events involving them.

The school had also been keeping behavioral data for three years on one behavior: head contacts (to tables, knee, wrist, etc.). The data from the year prior to the intensive SI program was in a differ-ent form that could not be meaningfully compared. However, the data during the two years of therapy were directly comparable and the fall term data are shown in Tables 2 and 3. The transition year, 1984-85, illustrates extreme fluctuations in behavior from day to day as well as peaking after school holidays. Both of these observa-tions had been reported by school staff in years past. The 1985-86 data show a much lower, steadier graph with no peaks above 60 incidences, compared with days of over 200 head contacts the pre-vious year.

The school psychological evaluation, mandated every three years, was done in October 1985 and independently reflected many of D's changes. Testing results were reported at the same intellec-tual level but indicated that D had a wider range of applications, behaviors and skills at that level, was less involved with many of his habitual behaviors, and was performing more on task.

Family

The family objective of being able to enjoy D more and integrate him more fully into their lives is being achieved. The mother, who participated eagerly in his treatment, increased her number of weekly visits and eventually included D's sister more often as his hair pulling behavior decreased.

By December, 1985, the mother discovered that she could have D ride in the front seat of the car using only the regular car shoulder seat belt. Previously it had been necessary to elaborately restrain him with a harness in the back seat to preclude his self-release and typical destructive and distracting behaviors. D will respond appro-priately to a simple command for "good hands" if he reaches to interfere with the steering wheel or gear shift.

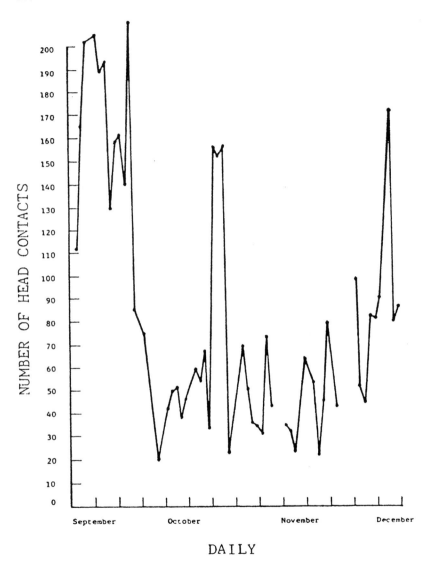

Table 2.   D's Head Contact Data
            Fall School Term 1984

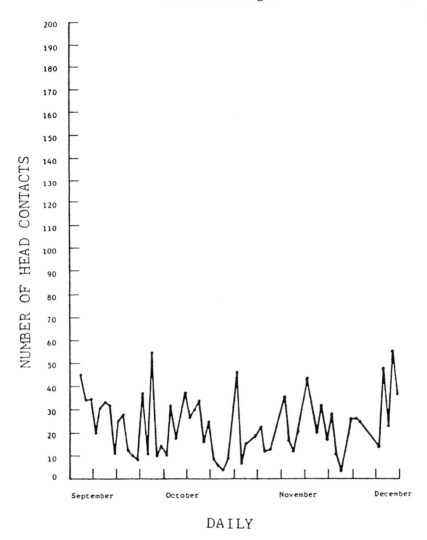

DAILY

Table 3. D's Head Contact Data
Fall School Term 1985

Dental Care

Another important result that reflects D's ability to cooperate and control his own behavior, and that also reflects an economic impact of therapy, is D's dental hygiene program. In the past, D had to be anesthesized for routine dental inspection and cleaning of his teeth. Because of the medical risk and the high costs this was only done every three years. Projected costs for 1985 were $2,000.00. In the spring of 1985 after ten months of occupational therapy utilizing a sensory integrative approach, and three months of an intensive oral stimulation-feeding program, a dentist willing to try to examine D without sedation was found.

D was cooperative with the examination, opening his mouth upon request and tolerating the exploration of his mouth. A cleaning appointment one month later was equally successful for a total cost of $35.00. A repeat dental check-up and cleaning was done in April of 1986.

DISCUSSION

Effect of the Oral Program

Special, additional expertise in oral-motor procedures played a key role and deserves emphasis. The intensive oral-facial stimulation and feeding program initiated by an experienced occupational therapist noticeably facilitated his sensory integration program.

In normal development, the oral region is one of the earliest organizers of motor, interpersonal/social and behavioral skills. One of the basic premises of a sensory integration approach is that the child must integrate his own system. Oral-motor activity was at an adaptive level of function within D's ability range. With the demand for goal-directed motor responses of sucking, chewing and swallowing built upon new sensory experiences, D may have been better able to organize his own system and integrate sensations and motor input. Parallel gains may then have been possible in other areas of functioning as adaptive responses were required and elicited in therapy, at school and in the group home.

The feeding program seems to have further benefited the sensory integration programming by providing a powerful motivational tool for sensory integrative activities. D was much more cooperative with sensory integrative activities when food was involved, not as a reward but as an integral part of the therapy activity e.g., sucking a thick yogurt shake through tubing while balancing in sitting on a big ball. The two programs were mutually reinforcing and created opportunities for skills to become automatic.

Impact of Other Services

It would also be appropriate in evaluating results to assess the impact of other disciplines, programs and care-givers. The major caregivers (family, group home and school personnel) were variables that were fairly constant. D had the same teacher for three years, including the year prior to intervention. D has also been in the same group home for over five years. While the location changed once during therapy and staff have rotated and changed rather frequently, the administration and the general philosophy directing the group home and its activities have been reasonably consistent.

The behavior management programs based upon behavior modification theory used both in the group home and at school have continued and appear to be more successful now. Moreover, these programs with their thoughtful, responsible expectations for behavior, have probably greatly enhanced D's achievement. Without the group home and school eliciting and encouraging higher levels of adaptive functioning, D's gains may not have been so solidly achieved.

Therapy Highlights

As D has improved, his therapy activities have expanded to use a greater variety of sensory integration modalities as well as allowing the use of other therapeutic techniques.

The initial therapy sessions involved offering selected sensory stimulation sources (vibrator, net, textures, weighted objects) and observing how D used them, what was or was not satisfying to him and then allowing him the time and space to use them as needed. This permission for him to direct the course of treatment based on his neurophysiological needs required a great deal of interpretation to group home staff, school and the family. The philosophy of co-operating *with* D and his observed needs rather than imposing activities and requiring him to conform to therapy demands was new to them. How this approach was therapeutic and did not give D carte blance to have his own way and manipulate others had to be demonstrated in light of some of the initial goals such as calming behavior, increasing attention span and making life around D more pleasant.

Therapy sessions six months later still found D spending long periods of time experiencing basic sensations although the equipment was more varied. For example, a vibrating table had been acquired and D could be encouraged to lie on it. It was with the vibrating table that total relaxation in a fully extended posture was first elicited. At the same time, he spent less time curled up with the hand held vibrator.

More active, adaptive response activities also had begun to emerge. He could be enticed into the suspended net although he usually preferred sitting or supine positions. For example, in sitting, D would reach for blocks in various planes and fit them into a three shape sorter can. The reaching precipitated movement experiences, and required postural adjustments as well as eliciting arm extension and head turning. On the scooterboard, he would sit and propel himself by walking his feet fifteen feet across the room to retrieve objects such as rings for stacking on a dowel.

The availability of the suspended net in the group home setting offered D the opportunity to occasionally self-select the net for gentle self-swinging and swaying in supine in the evenings. Group home staff were appreciative of its calming effects before meals or bedtimes.

With the integration of his oral-motor feeding program into his ongoing therapy, D was more easily directed into activities by incorporating food within the activity. D would swing prone in the net to reach for apricot or cheese morsels to put in his mouth, chew and swallow. He would willingly propel the scooterboard prone with his hands across the room to use his lips or tongue to get peanut butter dabs off a small flat plate held by another person. He could then be pulled by his legs or by his hands (sometimes with a rope) back across the room to continue the cycle.

By the third six month period, D's increased tolerance for hands on manipulation allowed the therapists to work more specifically on releasing tight muscle groups, and develop diagonal and rotational patterns. The addition of a platform swing facilitated this work during reaching and sorting activities as well as providing another means of offering vestibular input.

The school occupational therapist also began expanding D's oral-motor program with pursing and blowing activities in readiness for pre-speech sounds that had become new educational objectives.

The intensity of his supportive group home therapy sessions diminished over time, giving way to intermittent sessions of varying lengths of time that depended on the availability of the staff and D's wishes and needs.

Currently, in a clinic setting, D now swings himself prone in the net with good neck extension and will even spin himself three turns. He swings in straddle sitting, on a bolster swing (horse) with the therapist which provides her with an opportunity to increase freedom of movement in his pelvis and hips. D enjoys propelling himself prone on the scooterboard down a ramp to a target activity and can then be pulled back up the ramp with a rope to repeat the activity several times.

A current favorite activity is playing in a swimming pool of pinto beans. The therapist adapts this activity in a variety of ways. With D prone over the therapy ball and bearing weight on his hands and arms in the pinto beans, he enjoys playing with the beans, scooping and stirring which requires him to shift weight. The weight shifts and ball movement elicit continuous postural adjustments. Or, sitting in the beans, D enjoys pouring beans through long cardboard tubes which requires arm and neck extension as he also receives tactile input.

A vibrating pillow was also introduced to D and has become a new way in which D calms and reconstitutes himself in the classroom or other group situations after activities or when he becomes stressed. He has combined it with rocking in a rocking chair at school and also with sitting in a "bath" of hard plastic balls in his summer program.

Potential Danger

The potential danger for D is that care-givers may begin to expect too much from him. It has been so gratifying to see such major, important changes, that one could easily unrealistically expect him to continue to achieve at the same rate. If the demands to perform to external standards become too great, his behavior is likely to reveal the stress and lead to regression.

Will Gains Last?

Indications are that if the above precautions are observed, D should maintain his gains. The graphs certainly show that he maintained these levels of behavior for the better part of a year while still in therapy. There have been episodes in which behavior regressed although not to the levels prior to treatment. When tension in his environment and new pressures on him to behave in certain ways were alleviated, he quickly returned to highest levels of functioning.

Future Programming

In the initial evaluation, 2 to 3 years of therapy were suggested. D has completed two years of therapy. He is being continued in private therapy on a weekly basis although the locus has changed from the group home to a clinic setting that was only recently available.

Residual flexion persists in the legs during standing and walking and needs to be addressed. D also continues to demonstrate a strong need for tactile and proprioceptive input in and about the neck area. The program will also aim toward increasing play and manipulative skills as well as postural fluidity and pleasure in sensory play experiences.

It is expected that in the future, other programs will be able to meet D's maintenance needs in sensory motor areas. When direct treatment is reduced and eventually discontinued, the family may want occasional consultations to help them maintain the flow and direction of school and group home programming in order to preserve the sensory integration philosophy that helps people accept D at his level of functioning and understand his behavior in terms of neurophysiological needs.

SUMMARY

A case report on the evaluation, treatment and results of a sensory integration based occupational therapy program with a severely mentally retarded/autistic fifteen year old boy was presented. The facilitating effect of an oral stimulation and feeding program combined with the sensory integration program was assessed as well as the impact of other supportive care-givers. Concerns and future programming needs were briefly considered.

APPENDIX A

Highlights of the Oral Program

Oral-facial stimulation preceeded snack time with all stimulation moving towards a closed mouth. Aquarium tubing with an orthoplast lip seal was provided to encourage lip closure (not teeth biting) during straw drinking. Resistance to the sucking, for proprioceptive input, was provided through thickened drinks such as yogurt shakes.

To elicit combined cheek and tongue action, small pinches of cereal were deposited between gums and cheeks. Bite-chew sequences were encouraged by the use of strips of cheese, beef jerky, apple or dried apricot placed between the side teeth. The strips were advanced slowly to provide constant stimulus biasing D's tongue to the side as he bit and chewed repeatedly. Three to four strips were provided to one side then repeated to the other side.

In order to help these activities in the mouth become more automatic and to integrate oral motor skills with whole body activities, sucking/drinking and chewing activities were combined with balance and movement by having D sit and respond to gentle movement on a therapy ball or platform swing.

An April update to the program (one month after program began) was the addition of a cap with a 3/4 inch elastic jaw strap to be worn during the first three-quarters of the snack time to "alert" the jaw for the last one-quarter of time without it.

Using Sensory Integration Principles with Regressed Elderly Patients

Mary A. Corcoran, MA, OTR/L
Donna Barrett, OTR

SUMMARY. Sensory deprivation in the elderly is an acquired syndrome which responds to intervention based on sensory integration principles and a sensitivity to former roles and cultural influences. Clinical observations of a group of regressed nursing home residents revealed maladaptive responses similar to those described by King in a sample of non-paranoid schizophrenic patients. Observations of maladaptive behavior were noted in posture and motor activity, perception, communication, cognition and psychosocial behavior. In the demonstration project presented here, eleven nursing home residents displaying symptoms of sensory deprivation were randomly assigned to one of two groups, intervention or control. The control group participated in individualized treatment utilizing biomechanical principles. In the intervention group, sensory integration principles provided the framework in a program which structured the environment to promote adaptive responses. The groups met for forty minutes twice weekly during a sixteen week period. A pretest-posttest comparison revealed significant improvement in the adaptive responses of the intervention group.

In response to the many studies on sensory deprivation, Ayres[1] concluded that the ability to cope with the environment can diminish in the absence of an adequate stream of stimuli. Due to a combination of normal age-related sensory changes and pathological con-

Mary A. Corcoran is currently employed as an instructor in the Department of Occupational Therapy, College of Allied Health Sciences, Thomas Jefferson University, Philadelphia, PA. She also practices as an independent contractor specializing in gerontic occupational therapy. Donna Barrett is employed as a staff occupational therapist with the Lutheran Home at Moorestown, NJ.

This article appears jointly in *Sensory Integrative Approaches in Occupational Therapy* (The Haworth Press, 1987) and *Occupational Therapy in Health Care*, Volume 4, Number 2 (Summer 1987).

ditions which frequently occur in the elderly, many older people experience sensory deprivation. Correlations between many "general effects" and sensory deprivation have been noted in institutionalized geriatric patients.[2] These effects are identified as disorders of thinking and concentration, drifting of thought, disorientation in time, body illusions and delusions, complaints of restlessness, somatic discomforts, paranoid-like delusions, hallucinations and images, and emotional reactions such as anxiety.

O'Neil and Calhoun[3] postulate that normal peripheral sensory loss has a causal effect on cognitive and/or behavioral deterioration. They found that multiple sensory losses had a significant negative correlation with a mental status evaluation score in nursing home residents who are mobile. This result highlights the crucial role of adequate environmental stimulation, especially in individuals who are sensory restricted as well as immobile. In the presence of a condition of sensory deprivation, an older person's environmental coping process becomes dysfunctional and responses to sensory input become maladaptive.

ADAPTIVE RESPONSES IN THE PRESENCE OF SENSORY DEPRIVATION

Adaptive responses are the end product of a process by which the central nervous system takes in information, interprets it, and produces meaningful action. Responses may be affective, motoric, physiological or functional alterations. In 1974, Lazarus presented a multivariate analysis of factors mediating the elderly's adaptive responses to sensory input.[4] The analysis offers perception of threat and resultant stress as intervening factors between environment and behavior. If a stimulus is appraised as a threat, the individual's coping mechanisms are scanned for an appropriate response to the threat. When the appraisal process, a function of cognition, is faulty due to sensory deprivation, stimuli normally perceived as nonthreatening become stressors. The resultant response is labeled as maladaptive behavior.

King's application of sensory integration to institutionalized nonparanoid schizophrenic patients further connects sensory perception, integration and physiologic stress responses.[5] She utilized sensory integration techniques to address performance deficits in cognition, communication, affect, bilateral movements, praxis, posture and activity level. Participants in King's program evidenced more adaptive responses in such areas as appearance, sociability and task behavior.

SENSORY INTEGRATION PRINCIPLES GUIDE INTERVENTION IN GERIATRICS

Ayres and King laid the theoretical basis for techniques developed by Ross and Burdick[6] to address the maladaptive responses of regressed psychiatric and geriatric patients. These authors published the results of an intervention method utilizing sensory integration principles during daily sessions that were comprised of five stages. These stages moved linearly from alerting activities involving tactile, kinesthetic and proprioceptive input to graded opportunities for organized thought and behavior. The five components are outlined below.

Stage One: This stage opens the session with a welcoming activity and establishes some continuity with the previous group session. It utilizes tactile input to alert and set the emotional tone.

Stage Two: This component converges sensory input in the premotor cortex and encourages gross motor movement and proximal joint co-contraction patterns. Stage two facilitates improvement in body scheme, posture, and muscle balance during activities designed to provide vestibular, proprioceptive and tactile input.

Stage Three: This stage influences the thalamus and cortex to modify and correlate all sensory information. The selective sensory stimulation is then facilitated to conscious awareness through a stage three activity.

Stage Four: This component organizes thoughts and behavior.

Stage Five: This closing stage establishes continuity with the future and reaffirms the emotional tone of the session.

The principles of sensory integrative theory provide the foundation of Ross and Burdick's techniques. Tactile, vestibular and proprioceptive stimuli are effective in alerting the individual due to the basic information relayed to the reticular activating system, limbic system and cranial nerves. Visual information is given meaning through association with what is experienced in movement and in touch. Auditory input is processed with the assistance of vision, and the culmination of meaningful sensations helps to form abstract and cognitive thoughts.[1]

Occupational therapists who employ Ross and Burdick's method of intervention with geriatrics will utilize techniques similar to traditional occupational therapy utilizing a sensory integrative approach. Therapists should note, however, that although their clients exhibit symptoms of sensory integrative disorders, they do not have the same needs as patients typically involved in programs employing sensory integration procedures. Most elderly persons with histories of competent occupational performance may be assumed to possess adequate foundations of sensory processing skills. Their lack of age and culturally appropriate responses cannot be attributed to a developmental sensory integrative problem, but rather to deprivation of sufficient stimuli needed to perpetuate adaptive functioning. Sensory integrative disorders are commonly regarded as innate delays in development of neural interconnections. Ayres[1] states that sensory integrative activities facilitate processing of sensations which have never been integrated before. She postulates that the brain replaces some sensory-motor activities with mental and social responses as it matures. Therefore, remediation with patients who have already acquired the developmental groundwork for more complex neural functioning begins with sensory-motor activity to strengthen neural interconnections, but does not remain predominantly motoric. Intervention will instead emphasize more age appropriate mental and social adaptive responses.

PROGRAM DESCRIPTION: PROMOTING ADAPTIVE RESPONSES IN REGRESSED NURSING HOME ELDERLY

Overview of the Program

In 1985, a group of eleven nursing home residents participated in a sixteen week intervention program to improve general and task behavior. The eleven residents were identified by nursing staff as their most "regressed" patients. All identified residents were female, although no criteria was established regarding the sex of the participants. Six residents were randomly selected to become members of a group based on principles of sensory integration. The five additional residents received biomechanical intervention according to individual treatment needs. Both groups were seen by the occupational therapist twice weekly for forty minutes.

The eleven group participants were evaluated by an occupational therapist who was blind to treatment group assignments. The evaluator utilized the Comprehensive Occupational Therapy Evaluation (COTE) to rate twenty-five behaviors in areas of general, interpersonal and task skills.[7] Each behavior was rated from zero to four based on the severity of the problems, and each is thought to be important to adaptive functioning in an individual's environment. The results of the COTE administration, combined with clinical observations, disclosed maladaptive responses in five areas: posture and motor activity, communication, perception, cognition and psychosocial behavior.

Characteristics of the Sample

The characteristics of the sample are organized according to the five observed responses outlined above.

Observation of Posture and Motor Activity: Seventy percent of the population were bound by a flexed posture due to weak head, neck and trunk extensors. The entire group also demonstrated a paucity and decline in performance of automatic postural responses and an initial overall endurance for activity of approximately two minutes. All but two of the eleven participants received a score of moderate to severe interference with competence due to hypoactivity. The remaining two were observed to engage in hyperactive behavior. Eight were non-ambulatory and unable to propel a wheelchair. All group members exhibited a deficit in bilateral movements and seventy-five percent demonstrated severe problems in hand function. Poor hand function was exacerbated by unmanaged rheumatoid arthritis and spasticity.

Observations of Perceptions: The clinical picture of the eleven participants included varying degrees of deficits in visual tracking, left/right discrimination, and body part awareness. The entire population sought tactile input, and pursued opportunities for any stimulation, whether noxious or pleasant. All were minimally to severely apraxic and demonstrated psychomotor retardation. Additionally, seven members evidenced ataxia, and six exhibited signs of unilateral neglect.

Observations of Communication: All group members suffered from auditory problems and information reflecting the apparent severity of the deficits was not found in their medical records. Verbalization was usually reduced to one or two word responses following direct probing. Three participants, however, made no attempt at verbalization. Body language ranged from restricted to absent.

Observations of Cognition: COTE scale scores indicated that all participants engaged in moderately to severely impaired task behavior. Task behavior categories on the assessment consisted mostly of cognitive skills. Noted to be especially problematic were performances in the subsections of problem solving, decision making, reality orientation and attention span.

Observations of Psychosocial Behavior: The majority of group members were unable to socialize with peers or staff, even when directly approached. They evidenced no autonomy in interpersonal situations. All members presented either a flattened or inappropriate affect. They indicated an inability to take advantage of opportunities to constructively express their emotions.

Treatment Strategy

The intervention group used Ross and Burdick's techniques which were previously outlined.[6] The techniques were enhanced by a structured environment of graded activities, life review and group support. By allowing the elderly participant to respond to the structure of the environment, this total approach promoted competence and an attempt to regain an internal locus of control. Self esteem improved as individuals began to make choices about occupations based on personal values, roles and interests. A sample session is described below.

Stage One: Double handshakes were used during member introductions and orientation with a large calendar.

Stage Two: Various sized beachballs were utilized as each participant threw a ball to another member, while calling out that person's name, or their own favorite foods.

Stage Three: Hand-over-hand assistance was used during cutting and pasting of colorful, magazine pictures onto the group's seasonal collage. (The autumn collage consisted of pictures chosen by the group members which reminded them of that season.)

Stage Four: Each member identified the picture she had chosen for the collage, and stated why it reminded her of the autumn season. The therapist employed life review to stimulate discussion of characteristics of the autumn season, such as Halloween treats and cold weather. Life review is also used to integrate the past with the present in order to improve self esteem.

Stage Five: After identifying the date of the next session, the therapist served apple cider and ended the group by assisting members to pass handshakes.

The control group was based on rehabilitation of performance deficits affecting daily living skills. Therapeutic activities designed to improve strength, coordination, perceptual-motor skills and cognition were carried out in a group setting. Although group members participated in many sensory-motor activities, the sessions did not follow the five stage technique to promote increasingly complex mental and social responses. Additionally, techniques such as life review and facilitation of group support were not incorporated into the structure of the group. Examples of control group activities include arts and crafts involving gross and fine motor skills and self range of motion.

Results

Participants in the intervention group evidenced substantial clinical improvement in adaptive behavior at the termination of the program. No change was noted in the control group. Clinical results of the intervention group will be discussed using the five categories of observed behavior introduced earlier.

Observations of Posture and Motor Activity: The original members of the target population, previously hindered by a flexed sitting posture, made notable gains in head, neck and trunk extension. Several non-involved staff members remarked that they had never seen the patients sit so erect. All participants improved in automatic postural responses such that they could participate in the graded activities of the intervention group. Overall endurance for activity increased from an averge of two minutes to forty minutes. Hypoactivity and hyperactivity scores initially fell within the moderate to severe impairment range of the COTE scale. Following intervention, activity levels evidenced a positive gain of one interval on the scale.

Bilateral movements and hand skills became increasingly functional, although the majority of physical limitations were irreversible. Members with previously non-functional hands remained poor in hand function, but were noted to make more frequent attempts to use their hands.

Observations of Perceptions: Incidences of psychomotor retarda-

tion were substantially reduced in all group participants by the end
of the intervention period. Participants required less hand-over-
hand guidance, and half were able to motor plan sufficiently to lead
the group in a stage two activity. Left/right discrimination, as well
as body part awareness, became functional for the demands of the
structured intervention tasks. There was also a generalized reduction in unilateral neglect.

Observations of Communication: All group members displayed a
significant improvement in initiation of verbalization and quality of
verbal responses. One member, who was initially uncommunica-
tive, began to speak in one to two word sentences. Group members
turned and faced speakers and self expression was augmented by
facial and body movements. They initiated more verbal interactions
and often verbally comforted or supported each other. Verbalizations became more appropriate during group activities.

Observations of Cognition: The enhancement of cognitive skills
was reflected in a statistically significant improvement in task behavior scores recorded on the COTE posttest. Attention improved
from an approximate span of one or two minutes to fifteen minutes.
Each participant was able to maintain this level of attention as long
as the occupational therapist worked with her one-to-one or in a
group. She could not, however, maintain her attention to the task
while the therapist gave one-to-one assistance to another individual.
All group members began to recognize and solve simple problems
with minimal assistance at the end of the sixteen week intervention
period. Direction following moved from competence for only very
simple one-step, verbal and demonstrative directions to competence
for simple, two-step, verbal directions with an occasional need for
visual demonstration. By the termination of the program, each
group member was oriented to season, purpose and general format
of the group, and therapist's name. Although the majority were unable to recall other group members' names, each participant demonstrated visual memory of those who were part of the group.

Observations of Psychosocial Behavior: At the midpoint of the
intervention program, it was noted that the entire group began to
respond appropriately to shared experiences. For instance, the participants experienced episodes of "the giggles" when humorous
events occurred. Group members verbally, and on occasion, tacti-
lely comforted or supported each other. Affect, as well as verbalization, appeared to be more appropriate during treatment sessions. At

the termination of the program, intervention group members were noted to laugh and smile following pleasant stimuli and on a more frequent basis.

DISCUSSION

This demonstration project utilized a treatment technique, framed by sensory integration principles, which addressed the acquired problems of sensory deprived elderly people. The technique employed life review, graded activities, and group support in an environment of controlled sensory input. Further, it progressed the group members from physical interaction with sensory stimuli to graded oportunities to make age and culturally appropriate responses.

The project predicted that elderly, regressed patients who received the aforementioned treatment, would establish the performance foundations for more functional task skills. Expected rudimentary skills included general orientation, basic cognitive ability, improved endurance for activities, gross motor coordination and primary motor planning. However, results of pre- and postevaluation, including clinical observations, far exceeded original predictions. Additional adaptive behaviors, such as automatic postural responses, more normal activity level, perceptual-motor skill, self-expression, appropriate affect and social awareness were elicited.

Sufficient data has not been gathered to make recommendations for the global use of this technique. Additional questions are raised in the exploration of a sensory integration framework in geriatrics. What are the long term effects of its use on competencies in the elderly? If the benefits are short-lived, can this intervention be continuously implemented in the present health care delivery system? Finally, what modifications and refinements are necessary to improve its effectiveness in the promotion of occupational role functioning? Future avenues for research into the effects of sensory integration principles with geriatric populations are indicated.

There is a real need for effective methods of improving and maintaining competence levels in the growing number of elderly who suffer from sensory deprivation due to a combination of normal aging, physical inactivity and social isolation. Occupational therapists possess the theoretical background with which to provide this type of geriatric rehabilitation. Their utilization of sensory integration principles can be part of a total approach to prevent unnecessary institutionalization and loss of independence, as well as counteract the negative effects of sensory deprivation. Gerontic occupational therapists should consider verifying the findings of this project, as well as other demonstrated and research approaches within their practice arenas.

REFERENCES

1. Ayres J: *Sensory Integration and the Child*. Los Angeles: Western Psychological Services, 1979

2. Erber JT: The institutionalized geriatric patient considered in a framework of developmental deprivation. *Hum Dev* 22:165-79, 1979

3. O'Neil PM, Calhoun KS: Sensory deficits and behavioral deterioration in senescence. *J Abnorm Psychol* 84:579-82, 1975

4. Lazarus R: Response of the elderly to the environment: a stress-theoretical perspective. In *Aging and the Environment*, MP Lawton, Editor. New York: Springer Publishing Co., 1982

5. King LJ: A sensory integrative approach to schizophrenia. *Am J Occup Ther* 28(9): 529-36, 1974

6. Ross M, Burdick D: *Sensory Integration*. Thorofare, NJ: Slack, Inc., 1981

7. Brayman SJ, Kirby TF, Misenheimer AM, Short MJ: Comprehensive occupational therapy evaluation. *Am J Occup Ther* 30(2):94-100, 1976

The Use
of Computer-Assisted
Behavior Observation
in Sensory Integration Practice
and Research

Mary L. Schneider, MS, OTR
Maribeth Champoux, MS
R. Hannes Beinert

SUMMARY. In the past, occupational therapists have relied upon either indirect reports of client behavior or outcomes of standardized test paradigms to assess the efficacy of their treatment. The use of direct behavioral observations is proposed as an aid in the sensory integrative therapy process. Utilizing this method allows the therapist to quantify data, to devise and answer specific research questions, and to assess the progress of clients in treatment. Advice is given on how to best establish a behavior taxonomy to meet specific needs of the research or therapy situation. The benefits and drawbacks of computer-assisted direct behavioral observation are examined. It is concluded that computer-assisted direct behavioral observation could and should provide a valuable data collection tool in the occupational therapist's repertoire.

The observation of behavior is a central component in the evaluation and treatment of individuals requiring occupational therapy services. This is true in all areas of practice. In the sensory integrative approach, the accuracy of the evaluation and the efficacy of the

Mary L. Schneider and Maribeth Champoux are doctoral candidates, Department of Psychology, University of Wisconsin, Madison, WI 53706; Harlow Primate Laboratory, Madison, WI 53715; and Laboratory of Comparative Ethology, NICHD, Bethesda, MD 20205. R. Hannes Beinert is a software consultant at the Harlow Primate Laboratory, Madison, WI 53715.

This article appears jointly in *Sensory Integrative Approaches in Occupational Therapy* (The Haworth Press, 1987) and *Occupational Therapy in Health Care*, Volume 4, Number 2 (Summer 1987).

treatment are dependent on the shrewd observations of the therapist. Although computers have not traditionally been utilized in the mainstream of clinical practice, their growing potential promises to offer occupational therapists a valuable tool to enhance their skills as observers of behavior. Indeed, computers can actually improve the accuracy and consistency of the collected behavioral data while allowing the therapist to do so with greater ease and speed. Once observations have been recorded in this manner they can be easily translated into quantitative information that can be used for both descriptive purposes and for testing specific research hypotheses. These analyses in turn are of direct benefit to the client.

THE IMPORTANCE OF BEHAVIORAL OBSERVATIONS IN SENSORY INTEGRATIVE TREATMENT

In the sensory integrative treatment process,[1] the child is actively engaged in efforts to organize and structure his behavior and his environment. This process involves a dynamic interaction between the child and the therapist. More specifically, the therapist attempts to continually modify the environment so that the child's efforts to actively reorganize his behavior can be maximized. This process requires that the therapist constantly assess the transactions[2] between the child and his environment to determine whether adaptive integration is being facilitated or hindered. In essence, the process of therapy consists of a chain of events which is based on a complex reciprocity between the therapist and the child, which leads to a final outcome of improved organization of the child within its environment. The ultimate goal of therapy is that the improvement in the child's organization, based on neural integration and modification, will generalize to improved adaptation in the home, the school, and in social interactions. The efficacy of the treatment depends upon the ability of the therapist to observe the child's behaviors and appropriately modify the environment to elicit increasingly complex adaptive responses.

THE USE OF DIRECT BEHAVIORAL OBSERVATIONS IN THE TREATMENT PROCESS

Direct behavioral observations in occupational therapy can be used in a variety of settings, such as the classroom, the playground, and the sensory integration treatment setting. Quantifiable data from these situations can then be used to generate descriptive data or to answer specific research questions. Armed with descriptive data, one can begin to answer questions regarding the developmental processes that occur during the chain of events which comprise sensory integrative therapy. Answers to these questions could have implications for improving the effectiveness of treatment.

In addition to generating descriptive data, direct behavioral observations can be used to ask more specific research questions. Some examples of questions which would be amenable to this type of analysis include:

> Is there a relationship between a sudden increase in the duration of time spent in adaptive behavior in therapy and positive reports concerning behaviors at home or in school?

> Do children with different types of sensory integrative dysfunction follow different developmental sequences in therapy depending on the type of dysfunction?

> Are there differences in positive classroom behaviors between children engaging in sensory integrative therapy and their untreated counterparts?

AN EXAMPLE OF DIRECT BEHAVIORAL OBSERVATION IN THE SENSORY INTEGRATIVE TREATMENT PROCESS

To investigate the efficacy of sensory integrative treatment on behavior in the classroom, the therapist would initially devise a behavioral taxonomy for use in this particular situation. Relevant behaviors might include: purposeful activity, small motor fidgeting, gross motor squirming, vocalization, paying attention, not paying attention, passive staring off into the distance, etc. The therapist would then observe the child in the classroom at preordained times throughout the course of treatment. S/he would sit quietly at the back of the classroom and record behaviors for a predetermined amount of time using a computerized behavioral observation system. Depending upon the particular computer program used, such a system would allow for recording of frequency of behaviors, duration of behaviors, sequencing, or simultaneity of behaviors. Some software packages include data storage and statistical analysis capabilities. Data would be collected on the child before, during, and following the sensory integrative therapy. Data could also be collected on children used as control subjects. This method of assessing the effectiveness of treatment enables the therapist to be acutely aware of the behavioral changes induced by the treatment process.

DEVELOPING A BEHAVIORAL TAXONOMY

The act of direct behavioral observation involves three components: an observer, an individual being observed, and a behavioral taxonomy. The role of the observer is to record and preserve a permanent record of all relevant behaviors performed by the subject or client in a given time period.[3] The measuring instruments are the eyes, ears, and judgement of the observer. The form of the behavioral taxonomy is influenced by a multitude of factors, including the observation setting, the research question being asked, and the form in which behaviors will be recorded. Before beginning to develop a taxonomy, one needs to define the questions being asked and the conditions under which answers to those questions will be most salient.[4]

The conditions under which the subjects are observed will affect which behaviors are considered for observation. For example, if one is observing a child in his classroom, it would be very difficult, if not impossible, to use a taxonomy which involves facial expressions, eye movements, etc. If, on the other hand, one is observing the child while in close proximity, such as during a standardized paper and pencil task, the behavioral taxonomy might consist of very subtle behaviors.

The research question asked will also affect the taxonomy. For example, if one is asking questions pertaining to stereotypies, then the behavioral taxonomy will include a variety of typical stereotypies. If, on the other hand, the research question concerns attention in the classroom, then the behavioral taxonomy will include behaviors reflecting attentional processes. Once the observation conditions and the research question have been established, the next step in developing a behavior taxonomy involves simply watching the subjects and compiling a list of all the behaviors considered relevant in the particular situation. During this phase the boundaries of behaviors need to be delineated and the observer must decide what distinguishes one behavior from another. This can pose a particular problem for the occupational therapist involved in sensory integrative treatment, since some behaviors have discrete onsets and offsets while others have less definite boundaries.[4] When, for example, does a particular activity become classified as an adaptive response? Since one of the chief outcomes of improved sensory integration is manifested in the adaptive response, the investigator must be able to make fine distinctions between behaviors which may appear very similar. To do this, the observer should look for clues which signify the onsets and offsets of behavioral patterns. A shift in the orientation or the intensity of a child's behavior is usually a good indication that one behavioral unit is ending and a new one beginning.[4]

The final consideration in developing a behavioral taxonomy involves a decision regarding the form in which behaviors will be recorded. Behaviors can be viewed as being either states or events. Recording of states involves measuring the duration of behaviors. Events, on the other hand, are considered to be instantaneous occurrences, and the best way to record them is to collect data on frequency of onsets of behaviors.[5] More sophisticated scoring systems incorporate measures of simultaneity of behaviors and sequencing of behaviors. The interested reader is referred to Altmann[5] for a discussion of these issues.

THE UTILITY OF A COMPUTER-ASSISTED APPROACH TO DATA COLLECTION

Most traditional methods of recording behavioral data are compromises, as these methods are usually manual and hence limited by the abilities of the observer. Methods such as checklists allow recording of frequency of behavior but may lose information about the sequencing or the duration of the behaviors. Handwritten notes of ongoing behavior have a tendency to lag behind the action,[6] which may result in the loss of valuable data. Often the attention of the observer must shift back and forth between the action and the notebook, which results in a further data loss.[6] Voice tape recording and videotaping of ongoing behavior allow the observer to keep up with the action, but this necessitates a laborious and time-consuming transcription process.[6] Obviously, there are several advantages to a computerized data collection system. Depending upon the system, frequency, duration, and sequencing of behaviors are automatically recorded and computed. To duplicate this without a computer, an array of stopwatches, checksheets, and observers would be required. The computer can record data with much greater temporal accuracy than can the human observer. Behaviors can be recorded as they are ongoing, thereby avoiding the necessity of transcribing the data. The number of behaviors which can be recorded are limited only by the imagination of the observer. There are many computers on the market which are lightweight and portable, allowing for ease of data collection in any circumstance imaginable. Furthermore, some computer programs allow easy reduction and analysis of the collected data. In sum, the entire process of data collection is easier, quicker, and more reliable when computers are used.

LIMITATIONS OF DIRECT
BEHAVIORAL OBSERVATION

There are several limitations of observational research. First, this type of research can be costly both in terms of the demands on the time of the trained observers as well as the cost of the computer and software. In addition, the presence of an observer in a classroom or therapy session may actually influence the subject's behavior.[7] Finally, the fully trained observer functions as a switch, recording the onsets and offsets of the ongoing behaviors. Unfortunately, a certain amount of error is unavoidable as long as human beings are conducting the observations. One of the goals of the individual developing the behavior taxonomy is to attempt to minimize the occurrence of these errors. There are several methods to reduce the error inherent in this type of data collection. The individual devising the taxonomy must clearly define the behaviors and restrict the number of complex discriminations required by the observer. It is also necessary that interobserver reliability be high, and that observer error be spread across all experimental conditions.[8]

All the aforementioned problems along with a few extra are inherent in the use of computer-assisted behavioral observation. Computers can be costly and require training to use. Mechanical breakdowns can and do occur, although in our experience computer breakdown is less frequent than breakdown of our mechanical scoring machines. Computers require a power source, either batteries or electricity, and can be less portable and less useful in rugged conditions (e.g., a playground on a rainy day) than are a simple pad and pencil. Nonetheless, it is obvious that the advantages of a computer-assisted data collection system far outweigh the disadvantages.

IMPLICATIONS AND CONCLUSIONS

The computer-assisted behavioral observation method is potentially useful to occupational therapists working in the area of sensory integration treatment as well as in other areas of practice. This method has been gaining increasing respectability in many fields involved in developmental research and it has a great deal to offer occupational therapy. The potential usefulness of the method depends on several factors. The first is the willingness of occupational therapists to risk expanding into a new area of increasing sophistication. While computers are used in some areas of practice, they have not been incorporated into the mainstream of clinical practice. The second factor is that the benefits to be realized from this method depend upon the sophistication, creativity, and rigor of the occupational therapists. Occupational therapists are increasingly utilizing single-subject designs to evaluate treatment efficacy.[9] The computer-assisted behavioral observational method could provide a valuable tool for data collection in this type of design. And finally, the potential of this method depends on the ability of clinicians and researchers to work together. It has the potential for not only increasing the respectibility of occupational therapy, but also, more importantly, for improving the quality of the services we provide to our clients.

REFERENCES

1. Ayres AJ: *Sensory Integration And Learning Disorders*. Los Angeles: Western Psychological Services, 1972

2. Sameroff AJ: Early influences on development: Fact or fancy? *Merrill-Palmer Quarterly*, 21, 267-294, 1975

3. Sackett GP: Measurement in observational research. In G. P. Sackett (Ed.), *Observing Behavior, Vol II, Data Collection and Analysis Methods*(pp. 25-43), Maryland: University Park Press, 1978

4. Rosenblum LA: The creation of a behavioral taxonomy. In G. P. Sackett (Ed.),*Observing Behavior, Vol II, Data Collection and Analysis Methods* (pp. 15-24), Maryland: University Park Press.

5. Altmann J: Observational study of behavior: Sampling methods. *Behaviour, 49*, 228-265, 1974

6. Stephenson GR, Smith DB, and Roberts TW: The SSR system: An open format event recording system with computerized transcription. *Beh Res Meth Instr, 7*, 497-515.

7. Thorndike RL, and Hagen EP: *Measurement and Evaluation in Psychology and Education: Third Edition*. New York: John Wiley & Sons, 1969

8. Sackett GP, Ruppenthal GC, and Gluck J: Introduction: An overview of methodological and statistical problems in observational research. In GP Sackett (Ed.) *Observing Behav-*

ior, Vol. II, Data Collection and Analysis Methods (pp. 1-14), Maryland: University Park Press, 1978

9. Ottenbacher K, and York J: Strategies for evaluating clinical change: Implications for practice and research. *Am J Occup Ther, 38,* 647-659, 1984

The Clinician as Advocate for Sensory Integration

Barbara E. Hanft, MA, OTR/L

SUMMARY. This paper discusses professional advocacy as a means to promote occupational therapy services for clients. Although sensory integration is the focal point, the process discussed below for evaluating a system is valuable for promoting any aspect of occupational therapy. Examples of providing occupational therapy to children in a public school setting are used to illustrate the principles of the process.

The current environment of cost containment in health care demands that therapists look beyond clinical issues, and familiarize themselves with the external forces that define their practice. It is no longer possible to treat clients effectively while ignoring changes in reimbursement, health and education policy, and increasing competition from other providers.[1]

Occupational therapy personnel have traditionally viewed themselves as advocates for their clients, helping them attain new skills or regain those lost through disease or trauma. Today's practitioner must also promote their unique contributions to the client's well being if they are to remain viable partners in today's service arena. Approximately 75% of occupational therapy practitioners identify

Barbara E. Hanft currently works in the Government and Legal Affairs Division of The American Occupational Therapy Association, Inc. (AOTA) and is on the faculty of Sensory Integration, International. Her MA is in Counseling Psychology and she has 12 years experience as a pediatric occupational therapist in varied settings, including the public school system.

The author gratefully acknowledges the editorial assistance of Roland McDevitt, PhD, in preparing this paper.

This article appears jointly in *Sensory Integrative Approaches in Occupational Therapy* (The Haworth Press, 1987) and *Occupational Therapy in Health Care*, Volume 4, Number 2 (Summer 1987).

themselves as primary care providers.[2] Imagine the positive impact if each practitioner could incorporate professional advocacy into her daily activities.

The effective advocate knows how to use information to promote her cause. She knows her subject backwards and forwards, and she knows her adversaries' arguments and viewpoints. This knowledge is an essential prerequisite for effective promotion. Moreover, the effective advocate defines a specific context for her issue and draws plausible parallels and logical relationships for her audience. Using these principles, she can persuade others to accept and promote her particular point of view.

Similarly, occupational therapy personnel who wish to promote sensory integration must understand their subject and present sensory integration within a context that colleagues and clients can understand. Advocacy for sensory integration revolves around the following two premises, which are central to placing the subject within its context.

The first premise is that the clinician must thoroughly understand sensory integration theory and practice. The greater the therapist's knowledge of sensory integration, the greater her ability to advocate its benefits. This means, at a minimum, understanding how sensory integration compares with other professional frames of reference, such as neurodevelopmental therapy, perceptual-motor training and occupational behavior. For example, it is essential that the clinician distinguish sensory integration treatment from "sensory stimulation" and "vestibular input."

The second premise is that the context for sensory integration is occupational therapy. Occupational therapists facilitate adaptive responses to help people achieve mastery in age appropriate roles. In the context of sensory integration therapy, specific sensory input is carefully chosen to facilitate a somatomotor adaptive response which enables the individual to respond appropriately to the environment. Occupational therapy personnel use sensory integration as one of many treatment modalities, choosing the appropriate modality to meet the individual needs of each client.

In promoting sensory integration services, therapists usually face one of two situations. Either colleagues and other providers know very little about sensory integration and are noncommittal, or they have definite opinions which can be positive but often are extremely negative. In order to promote and expand services, changes must take place. Advocacy then becomes synonymous with change.

In order to effectively promote sensory integration services, the therapist must understand a three-step-process for implementing change:

1. analyze the situation to define the issue,
2. develop a strategy to target decision makers,
3. implement the strategy and assess effectiveness.[3]

The following are examples from a public school setting to illustrate this process.

ANALYZE THE SITUATION

Analyzing the situation is very similar to completing an activity analysis or client evaluation. It forms the basis for intervention and gives direction to actions promoting sensory integration. Rather than analyzing a specific action or individual set of strengths or weaknesses, look at your situation to determine what changes are needed to achieve your goal.

The first part of your analysis, then, is to clearly identify the ultimate goal. For example, your goal may be to extend occupational therapy services to include a sensory integration program, including classroom consultation, to public preschool classes for children with handicaps in your local school district.

Next, analyze the implications of your proposal from three perspectives: your own professional view, the client's and your employer's. Consider both the positive and negative effects of the proposed change in services so you can anticipate objections and promote the beneficial aspects of your program.

Exhibit I displays the diverse perspectives that might be anticipated in developing a sensory integration program for the public schools. Once you have considered these perspectives, you have an outline to present to your employer as well as to enlist support from others for your program. Consider your audiences' background and knowledge of sensory integration when choosing points to emphasize. This is crucial for being able to set the context for your audience so that he or she can relate to your message. Communicate using terms the audience understands.

When talking with parents emphasize that occupational therapy can help their children benefit from special education. Describe

EXHIBIT I

Impact of a Proposed Sensory Integration Therapy Program
in a Public School from Three Different Perspectives

Occupational Therapists and Assistants	Recipients of Services Parents, Children (and Educators)	School Administrators and Educational Staff
Positive Impact		
Increase awareness of occupational therapy and sensory integration	Help student benefit from educational instruction	Reduce costs by helping student function in least restrictive environment.
Promote collaboration with education and other related services staff	Improve functional skills of student	Provide consultation and training to educational staff.
Expand occupational therapy role and scope of practice	Modify behavior and enhance parent/ teacher/student interaction.	Provide a special service for diagnosis and treatment.
Negative Impacts		
Expand caseload	May lose classroom time.	Increase staff costs.
Increase administration and program planning (may detract from direct services).	Label student as needing special help.	Complicate scheduling of services.
		Cost of equipment/space.

how sensory integration can help a child acquire the basic motor and perceptual foundation needed for classroom activities. For example, if you are talking with parents of preschoolers, emphasize the child's need to know how to pick up one foot and put it into his pants leg while balancing on the other leg in order to get dressed. The child must have good feedback from his muscles and joints to tell him what's going on with his body. If the child is older and must complete written assignments, emphasize the tremendous organization needed to simultaneously direct the hand to form each letter, space it on the page, hold the pencil appropriately and decide what to say while ignoring the distractions from the hallway and playground.

Discussions with teachers and school administrators should emphasize the specialized consultation an occupational therapist trained in sensory integration can provide. A sensory integration evaluation can yield important data regarding sensory channels the student uses for learning. Special educators must adapt their teaching and incorporate specific activities for visual or kinesthetic learners. In addition, language therapists can incorporate tactile and motor activities in their sessions with dyspraxic children who have difficulty articulating ideas.

School administrators are interested in how specialized services can reduce costs by helping children function better in the school setting. Give examples of how a particular student's problem may prevent him from participating in certain aspects of the school program. Educating students in the "least restrictive environment" is a salient issue in the public schools and means that each exceptional student is educated in a setting which is appropriate to his or her individual needs. Sensory integration therapy coupled with classroom consultation can help a child with gravitational insecurity participate on the playground, in physical education sessions, as well as find a comfortable seating arrangement for academic tasks.

Analyzing the situation also requires you to identify the two different influences setting the stage for your proposal: the source of influence and the actual person(s) responsible for enforcement. The source of influence comes in the form of state or federal laws and regulations, school policies and employer attitudes, which all influence your work setting in pervasive ways (Exhibit II).

For example, federal law, P.L. 94-142 (Part B of the Education of the Handicapped Act), mandates occupational therapy services in the public school system *only* if the student needs these services to benefit from special education. Students with motor problems not requiring special education are ineligible for occupational therapy services despite an occupational therapist's assessment that improvement in functional skills can still be expected.

In developing a strategy for promoting sensory integration, knowing what you must modify, whether it be laws, attitudes and/or policies, will define the scope of your actions. It is far easier for the clinician to change school policy or the personal attitude of a principal when she comes in regular contact with the decision maker or decision making body that can exercise the authority to approve and support your program. If you do not possess the necessary authority to implement the desired change, you must determine if the decision makers are within your own immediate environment or at a re-

EXHIBIT II

Sources Which Can Influence a Proposal to Expand a Sensory Integration
Program in the Public Schools

Attitudes:	Beliefs and opinions formed by personal experience, generally unwritten and nonspecific. Example: Occupational therapists are not trained to work with exceptional children in the school system.
Policies:	Institutional procedures, either written or unwritten, which help govern a work setting such as a public school. Example: Only students with physical disabilities should receive occupational therapy.
Laws:	Acts of Congress or state legislatures which are approved or passed over the veto of the chief executive. Example: Education for the Handicapped Act (Part B of this Act is commonly cited as P.L. 94-142).
Regulations:	Description and translation of the generalities of law, carrying the force of law. Example: The Code of Federal Regulations contains specific sections regarding P.L. 94-142, such as the definition of occupational therapy and handicapping conditions.

gional, state or national level. Remember that your immediate supervisor may not be the decision maker responsible for the policy you would like to see changed.

Many times, however, you will find support for your program within your work setting from your local school board or director of special education and related services. These decision makers may have the authority to change policy to enable you to start your program immediately. When decision makers are removed from your work setting, making it difficult to deal directly with them, collaborative efforts become particularly important.

TARGETING THE DECISION MAKER

Once you have analyzed the situation and identified the decision makers, target them to receive information. This frequently involves building coalitions to enlist the aid of others who can support your position.

For example, Exhibit III illustrates a strategy for enlisting support

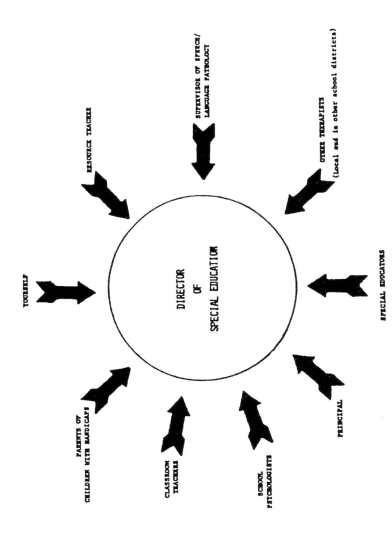

RESOURCE TEACHER

SUPERVISOR OF SPEECH/
LANGUAGE PATHOLOGY

OTHER THERAPISTS
(Local and in other school districts)

TEACHERS

DIRECTOR
OF
SPECIAL EDUCATION

SPECIAL EDUCATORS

PARENTS OF
CHILDREN WITH HANDICAPS

PRINCIPAL

CLASSROOM
TEACHERS

SCHOOL
PSYCHOLOGISTS

EXHIBIT III. Targeting the source

143

to influence your targeted decision maker, the local Director of Special Education and Related Services. The Director works closely with the Supervisor of Speech and Language Services and is also a personal friend of the resource teacher. These associates of the Director are potential allies in your efforts to persuade the Director that your program is worthy of support.

Moreover, the Director may have guidelines imposed by the State Education Agency regarding how occupational therapy services are provided within the state. Other clinicians in your state may be able to furnish you with examples of successful programs that comply with these guidelines.

Review the therapist, client and school perspectives of your proposed program (Exhibit I). What other groups or individuals would stand to benefit from your program? Parents of children with handicaps might be useful allies because they are clients of the public schools. Educators who have taught students with special needs could understand the special teaching strategies needed and might support direct service for the students, as well as consultation and inservice training for themselves. Once you have enlisted these allies, it is essential that they become well informed concerning the program you are advocating. If possible, enlist the support of parents and teachers who have had experience with sensory integration therapy. Just as you must be informed about your subject in order to promote it effectively, so must your support system.

IMPLEMENT YOUR STRATEGY

Once you identify the decision maker and organize a support system to promote your point of view, you can present your proposal. The timing and points of contact for presentation can be critical, so choose them carefully. Your efforts could be futile if you submit your proposal two days after the school board meets to review the budget for the next year. You must contact the decision maker in the appropriate time and manner. You would want to know whether you must attempt to modify a proposal that is in the working draft stage, or change a policy that has already been implemented. Talk to people who know the decision makers and the issues that concern them. Decision makers often listen to or depend on others in their own system for advice or counsel. Identifying these individuals and professional groups will help you target your coalition to help you lobby for your proposal.

Changing facility policy requires that you understand the decision making process within your organization. Perhaps your immediate supervisor has stipulated that all therapy will be delivered in a consultative format. Find out why your supervisor has taken this position. Is this a policy formulated by his supervisor or the state department of special education? To whose needs is he responding? What experience has your supervisor had with other service delivery options for occupational therapy such as monitoring and direct service?[4]

Once you understand why this policy was formulated, you can enlist supporters as illustrated in Exhibit III. You will also want to consider your approach for trying to persuade your supervisor to change his policy. Does he respond more favorably to a proposal in writing or presented orally? Which arguments are most likely to catch his attention: cost effectiveness, utilizing staff specialty areas, developing a model program or educating children with special needs? Can you propose a program which also will meet his goals?

As you implement your strategy, try to assess its effectiveness as you proceed. Follow-up is crucial throughout each of the three steps, but particularly during this stage. If you promise additional information, provide it. Follow telephone calls with memos or letters reiterating your points.

Encourage your supporters to make contact with decision makers and debrief them after they do. Find out whether you need to increase your support or ask them to "hold off" for awhile. Finally, thank your supporters for their help and keep them informed of events and decisions.

CONCLUSION

The process of influencing decision makers usually requires planning and effort, by more than one individual. But the power of each individual to influence colleagues and decision makers should not be underestimated. Even if you are not involved in a coordinated effort to change policies or programs, you can promote sensory integration by helping to establish positive attitudes regarding the profession of occupational therapy. Take the initiative to:

• Speak to local parent or professional groups regarding the benefits of occupational therapy and sensory integration.

- Organize inservice sessions or continuing education workshops on sensory integration for your staff and colleagues, and invite key members of other disciplines to attend as guests.
- Invite colleagues, administrators, politicians and influential consumers to attend an open house or "occupational therapy day" in your facility.
- Develop a fact sheet or brochure describing your services for visitors.
- Prepare yourself and your staff to speak extemporaneously to visitors about occupational therapy and sensory integration.
- Initiate a once-a-month interdisciplinary informal lunch where each professional speaks on specialized topics. Offer to give the first presentation on sensory integration.

Promoting change in the work setting is a logical extension of the practitioner's efforts to elicit adaptive behavior from clients. Becoming an effective change agent to promote sensory integration as a clinician requires analysis of the issue, targeting decision makers and building coalitions for support of a specific program. Although changing policies, laws and regulations usually requires a collaborative effort, the individual practitioner in her daily activities can be highly influential in changing and developing positive attitudes towards the profession.

REFERENCES

1. Christiansen C: Research: An economic imperative. The *Occup Ther J Res* 3(4): 195-198, 1983

2. Silvergleit I: Research and Evaluation Division of The American Occupational Therapy Association, Inc. Personal Communication, August 12, 1986

3. Scott SJ and Acquaviva J: *Lobbying for Health Care – A Guidebook for Professionals and Associations*. Rockville, Maryland: The American Occupational Therapy Association, Inc., 1985

4. American Occupational Therapy Association. *Guidelines for Occupational Therapy Services in the School System*. Rockville, Maryland, 1986

Improving the Work Potential
of Brain-Injured Adolescents
and Young Adults:
A Model for Evaluation
and Individualized Training

Ann V. Deaton, PhD
Cathy Poole, COTA
Denise Long, OTR

SUMMARY. Brain injured individuals have a unique set of skills and deficits which make them difficult to place in traditional jobs and work programs. Although they may function at a relatively high level intellectually, these individuals often demonstrate deficits in attention, motivation, memory, and social skills. A variety of strategies must be employed in assessing and developing the work potential of the brain injured individual. This paper describes a work program that has been designed to meet the unique needs of the brain injured population. Case examples are included to illustrate application of these strategies.

The authors are affiliated with Cumberland Hospital for Children and Adolescents, New Kent, VA.

This article appears jointly in *Sensory Integrative Approaches in Occupational Therapy* (The Haworth Press, 1987) and *Occupational Therapy in Health Care*, Volume 4, Number 2 (Summer 1987).

Little has been written about assessing the work potential and programming needs of brain-injured adolescents and young adults, although this population grows yearly. The present article is a description of how brain injuries affect work potential and how the resulting needs for prevocational assessment and specific training programs for brain injured persons can be addressed. The program described takes place in the context of an inpatient rehabilitation setting in a pediatric hospital. Throughout the paper there is an emphasis on the need for ongoing assessment, creative problem solving, and the acknowledgment of individual differences in this population.

The term "brain-injured patients" is used in this paper to include those with all types of acquired brain dysfunction due to traumatic head injuries, illnesses (e.g., meningitis), brain tumors, and other causes; injured individuals are referred to as "patients" because this program takes place in a hospital setting. A few case vignettes may illustrate the kinds of patients and challenges for work programming with whom we are working.

> *Case 1:* Anne, a sixteen year old, sustained brain damage as a result of a brain tumor and the subsequent surgery required to remove it. She is a friendly and neatly groomed individual who is subject to rapid mood changes and sudden sleep onset. Her distractibility, slowness, inability to estimate time, and low frustration tolerance all impact significantly on her potential for any productive work role.

> *Case 2:* Joey, 18, suffered an episode of anoxia which resulted in diffuse brain injury. He is a passive individual who requires numerous repetitions to even learn someone's name. Joey is generally unaware of his appearance or his work responsibilities and is likely to wait for someone to tell him what to do rather than initiating anything himself.

> *Case 3:* Pamela is a 20 year old who sustained a traumatic brain injury in a motor vehicle accident. As a result, she has severe memory and social skills deficits as well as impaired motor and sensory function on one side of her body. Pamela has a great deal of difficulty following instructions, but is motivated to improve her job skills and can function relatively well in a highly structured situation.

As these cases illustrate, a brain injury or illness can have a dramatic impact on vocational functioning and, in children and adolescents, on work potential. Any condition which affects the brain can affect virtually any area of functioning. This problem is becoming increasingly evident as improvements in medical technology have enabled more and more severely brain injured persons to survive. Since some readers may not be familiar with the range of abilities affected by brain injury, we will begin by discussing these. What makes working with brain-injured persons unique is that they are unlike many other groups of disabled persons in their pattern of strengths and deficits. Typically, these persons are not impaired in all areas but, rather, have retained some relative strengths which may be useful in compensating for deficits. One of the areas frequently affected by any kind of condition affecting the brain is what can be broadly termed "cognition." Cognition is multidimensional, encompassing the range of abilities from just being oriented in place and time to being able to effectively problem-solve or change one's approach to a task when task conditions change. To a certain degree, these abilities are organized in a hierarchy such that if one can solve problems, it can be assumed that abilities less complex than problem-solving are intact or that the individual has found a means of compensating for deficits.[1] Disruption of basic skills such as the ability to focus attention is likely to interfere with all areas of functioning, although some individuals with intact higher level skills are able to compensate for these deficits. The basically hierarchical organization of cognitive abilities has significant implications for pre-vocational training in that lower level skills, once acquired, can be built upon. Briefly, cognitive abilities may be affected by brain injuries and, in turn, affect work potential in the following ways:

1. Orientation: Disorientation in its most severe form causes confusion about where one is, what day or time it is, and what has happened to cause the present circumstances. Disorientation often remains a problem for patients, like Joey, who continue to be confused about the day of the week or whether it is morning or afternoon, resulting in difficulty performing any activity which requires an awareness of time or place (e.g., an inability to keep track of when one needs to arrive at work; inability to locate workplace);

2. Attention: Attentional problems may manifest themselves in a

number of ways: a patient may have difficulty focusing attention on essential versus unessential aspects of the environment, may be unable to sustain attention appropriately on a
given task, or may be easily distracted, as Pamela and Anne
are. All of these attentional problems result in performing
work both inefficiently and, usually, incompletely;

3. Memory: When someone like Joey is unable to remember
what the requirements of a job are from one day to the next,
what the last instructions given were, what one's coworkers'
and employer's names are, and so forth, clearly his memory
problems will interfere with work relationships and limit his
potential;

4. Sequencing: Sequencing skills are required in following
multistep directions as well as completing complex tasks.
Even tasks such as simple filing or collating and stapling papers, which appear relatively simple, may be difficult for
someone who has deficits in their ability to sequence;

5. Problem solving: Whether or not we think of it as problem
solving, most jobs involve making numerous decisions during
the course of every day, ranging from what to do when a piece
of equipment malfunctions to how to handle a change in routine. Responding appropriately to these situations requires the
cognitive flexibility to generate a number of alternatives, anticipate their consequences, and choose accordingly, a relatively high level cognitive skill. Not surprisingly, Anne, Joey,
and Pamela all have problems in this area. In addition to these
specific cognitive deficits, a generalized effect of a brain injury seems to be the increased effort required for all cognitive
tasks such that even previously automatic activities may actually produce a significant level of fatigue, resulting in lowered
productivity overall.

As devastating as the impact of cognitive losses may be, research
has shown that the social-emotional changes resulting from brain
injury may have an even more profound impact on post-injury functioning and are, as well, more distressing to both family members
and those who come in contact with the injured individual. [2,3,4] Some
of the more common difficuties in this area are disinhibition, emotional lability, decreased frustration tolerance, and temper outbursts. As is readily apparent in the following descriptions, problems in some of these areas can be so significant as to make a person

with many good cognitive and work skills essentially unemployable. On the other hand, if these problems are improved or handled effectively, the abilities of the person can be harnessed and directed towards a satisfying work role and improved self esteem. The ways in which deficits in these areas become problems in work situations can be illustrated as follows:

1. Disinhibition: When patients say and do whatever comes to mind without trying to inhibit inappropriate behaviors, their relationships with employers, customers, and coworkers suffer greatly. Disinhibition may take the form of sexual inappropriateness, silliness, etc., but whatever its form, is likely to make people uncomfortable and sometimes frightened about working with the injured individual;
2. Anger control: An inability to modulate the expression of anger is a relatively common problem in head injured individuals resulting sometimes in either verbal or physical aggression as well as an inability to process information until calm again. Such problems make it difficult for these individuals to work with others or to accept and utilize criticism and feedback effectively;
3. Frustration tolerance: Given that many tasks will be much more difficult after a brain injury, frustration is likely to occur often and, depending on a patient's tolerance, may result in his or her (like Anne) prematurely stopping work on tasks which can be mastered or giving up when something does not go precisely right;
4. Emotional lability: Frequent mood changes or consistently depressed or euphoric mood can result from brain injury and have a significant negative impact on work relationships as well as the ability to stay focused and persist at tasks.

Besides these specific changes, it is important to recognize that brain injured persons typically differ from other candidates for work programs in a number of ways. In comparison to others with catastrophic losses, it should be noted that cognition is usually left intact by the loss of a limb or by injuries resulting in paralysis. While this does not imply that there are not a great many adjustments to be made by these patients, it does suggest that they retain the cognitive resources which should facilitate adaptation.

In comparison to mentally retarded clients, the brain injured patient may once again share some similarities. However, a significant difference is that at one time the brain injured patient presumably functioned at a higher level. This has both positive implications in that there may be previously learned skills and knowledge which remain intact. However, it also presents problems in that one's entire self concept may need to change and self-esteem is inevitably threatened when someone has to adjust hopes and expectations downwardly. Knowing that one cannot now do something he or she could previously do is also frequently a source of great frustration to the brain injured patient.

ASSESSMENT

At Cumberland, A Hospital for Children and Adolescents, the goals of the prevocational training program are threefold: (a) to identify work potential given the patient's interests, intact abilities, and use of compensatory strategies; (b) to teach basic work behaviors (promptness, neatness, cooperation) which are generalizable to any work setting; and (c) to improve self esteem and realistic future planning. The program is based upon several principles: first, it must begin at the patient's current level and increase in its demands as the patient's abilities increase; second, work must be meaningful, not 'busy work' even if it is designed to teach a certain skill; and, finally, it is assumed that maximal functioning will probably depend on a combination of adaptations by the patient and by the setting. That is, it is considered essential for the therapist to identify ways in which the environment can be altered to promote better functioning.

In order to build upon the first of these principles, that of beginning at the patient's level, training starts with an initial assessment of strengths and deficits. The Jacobs Prevocational Skills Assessment has proven to be useful in this respect. Developed by Karen Jacobs, an occupational therapist, this non-standardized assessment battery was developed initially for a learning disabled population. It consists of fifteen informal tasks which yield information regarding functional abilities in a variety of performance areas (for a complete description, see Jacobs[5]). The standard administration of the assessment requires minimal special training, permits data recording in a simple and non-disruptive manner, and usually requires less than two hours to complete. The Jacobs also boasts a number of other practical advantages. Within individual tasks, there is a range of complexity. The tasks may also be readily adapted to meet physical and cognitive limitations so that information on abilities and not just deficits can be collected. Also important to patients' self esteem, the focus of each of the fifteen tasks is highly relevant to actual work situations. Finally, the nature and requirements of the tasks help to ensure a high level of interest and motivation for adolescents and are designed to be of limited duration so that attentional difficulties to not preclude success. The assessment also provides for evaluation of comprehension of written, visual, and verbal directions.

Actual tasks on the Jacobs include carpentry assembly, environmental mobility, money concepts, and office skills such as filing and using a telephone directory. Recording the information from these tasks is quick and easy. The tasks themselves, as well as the functions on which they are primarily dependent, are presented on a brief rating sheet which can be completed during the evaluation.[5] This one page summary sheet allows quick identification of skills and behaviors associated with performing a variety of tasks. The evaluator can simultaneously jot down important test behaviors and skills as well as degree of perseverance, motivation, and cooperation. Personal appearance and hand dominance can also be observed. In addition, the evaluator notes any modifications of task instructions or adaptive equipment utilized.

With continued use of the Jacobs in evaluating brain injured patients, we have developed our own expectations of performance and behavior on the varous tasks included in the battery. While most early adolescents of average ability can easily complete all these tasks, many who have sustained brain injuries have difficulties. Using an experiential framework along with the checklist from the evaluation, individualized training programs are planned to target areas which are consistently weak while also targeting the improvement of self esteem by relying on strengths. For example, a patient with poor sorting skills but good frustration tolerance and good use of written directions might be assigned a redundant sorting task and allowed to perform it with the aid of written instructions. As sorting skills improve, the form of instructions might become verbal instead of written to begin to target direction following skill rather than sorting skills per se. Thus, the goal is to both remediate deficits and to teach compensation through the use of relative strengths.

TRAINING IN THE WORKSHOP

Central to an individual's sense of self-worth is whether or not they feel their life has meaning. Certainly, with work being a major life role, its meaningfulness to each individual affects self-worth and attitude. The program at Cumberland Hospital is based on the philosophy that work must be purposeful, goal-oriented, and meaningful in itself and to the patient. Within the prevocational program, patients are paid for performing functional work tasks which are designed to facilitate the achievement of their individualized objectives. All tasks are designed to accommodate a wide range of levels of supervision. The lower end of the range is 1:1 supervision while the highest level is semi-independent work with minimal supervision. The many gradations of structure and supervision within the range are implemented based on the needs of the individual patient. The work tasks have also been selected because of the fact that they lend themselves well to modifications. Each patient may require task modifications specific to his/her limitations and abilities. A task analysis approach to a multi-step task enables tasks to be modified to ensure that lower functioning patients achieve success in task performance.[6]

The work program is flexible and varied. A variety of tasks are used to maintain interest and attention as well as to facilitate cognitive flexibility. Work tasks are recruited from within the hospital through both formal and informal communication channels. For example, a memo to all staff is distributed periodically requesting that staff examine their "routine" tasks such as xeroxing and filing and route them to the prevocational workshop if they seem appropriate as work tasks for the patients. Current jobs include watering the plants throughout the hospital, stamping charge slips for use by therapists in billing, and xeroxing articles and memos for staff. Other jobs specifically designed for the workshop include a paper recycling project, doing payroll for workshop attendees, acting as cashier at a patient store where patients can spend their tokens, points, and money to buy desired items, and keeping inventory on the computer for the patient store. The hospital does not do contract work for outside agencies, as this sort of commitment makes training less flexible and more geared to producing a product than to focusing on the process of how the patient can learn to perform a work task effectively.

In order to develop the skills desired and most effectively accommodate the various physical and cognitive limitations of our patients, a variety of environmental modifications and compensatory tools are utilized. A major environmental consideration is wheelchair accessibility. The arrangement and layout of furniture, equipment, and task materials is such that wheelchair patients can conveniently maneuver. Accessibility is assured by having the workshop laid out with ample space around each work area, having all tables at appropriate heights, and task materials and equipment within reach.

In keeping with the philosophy to have the environment simulate that of a real work situation, job cards and time cards are used. Job cards specify the particular work task to be performed. Time cards are provided and located just inside the entrance to the workshop where workers must sign their time in and time out beside the appropriate day and date printed on the card. If necessary, color coding is used on the time and job cards to designate days of work. A clock and a calendar are located above the time cards to assist patients in filling out the card. The job and time cards, clock, and calendar serve as compensatory as well as environmental tools. The importance of appropriate appearance on the job is also emphasized when patients report to their "job" in the workshop. As necessary, patients are asked to inspect their appearance in a mirror hung in the workshop. Then, appearance and necessary individual changes are discussed. For Joey, this was particularly helpful in increasing his awareness of his usually sloppy appearance and his pride in himself.

Maps are another example of both an environmental and compensatory tool for patients with difficulties in memory or spatial orientation. A diagram of the hospital layout is used to develop skills in map reading and following visual directions. Patients involved in a paper recycling project must follow maps to learn where they need to go to collect the boxes of paper to be recycled. As a compensatory tool, maps may be used in place of or in addition to written or verbal instructions.

To facilitate the performance of patients who have difficulty remembering or sequencing, written directions are posted throughout the workshop environment as a reminder of the sequential order in which a task must be completed. Just as maps can serve as compensatory tools, written instructions can allow compensation for deficits in recalling or understanding modeled or verbal instructions. Step by step written instructions also can decrease confusion and organizational problems because the steps of the task are so clearly specified. When neither written nor verbal directions are effective, patients are sometimes presented with a pictorial sequence of the steps involved in a task.

A means of allowing compensations for physical deficits is providing mechanical guides on some of the equipment used in the workshop. These provide an opportunity for successful task performance by patients with conditions such as tremors or visual difficulties who would otherwise be extremely frustrated by certain tasks even though they understood what they needed to do. In the workshop there are several such guides. Two are on an addressograph machine, one to properly align the charge slip to be stamped in the addressograph and the other a built in guide to align the charge card so that it cannot be misplaced. The cash register used in the patient store also has a mechanical guide with cutouts around each of the most frequently used keys.

Along with the self esteem and pride that come when patients are successful, there is a need for more tangible rewards for their work. As different types of treatment strategies are effective with some patients and not with others, so it is with the rewards or reinforcers for good job performance. Most patients are paid with Cumberland "patient dollars" which they can use to make purchases at the patient store. For others, a token system is used where, for example, a patient can receive a set number of tokens for demonstrating particular behaviors such as being on time, completing a task, and minimal socializing while on the job. Another means of reinforcement is to immediately reinforce stages of task performance by depositing coins into a transparent bank which the patient is able to see at all times. Finally, for those patients to whom money is not a meaningful or effective reward, concrete reinforcers such as stickers or candy bars are used.

Progress in the workshop is monitored using a Performance Checklist (available from authors) which we have developed. At the conclusion of each session the patient's performance in vocational readiness areas are reviewed using this checklist. The checklist is divided into seven major areas, each of which encompasses a progressive range of behaviors. For example, the first major area is work factors. Within this category, behaviors range from "coming to work willingly" to "tolerance/endurance." The checklist is completed by the therapist following each session in the workshop. Because it was designed to be a quick, easy to use tool, a simple + or − is used to record the presence or absence of the particular behavior. At the conclusion of each session, the checklist is presented to and discussed individually with those patients who are at a level where they can participate in this type of performance evaluation and discussion. This method is convenient for evaluating progress as well as identifying problem areas relative to individual treatment goals. Moreover, it is an important means of visual and verbal feedback for patients which, along with the concrete feedback of actual task performance, serves to increase patients awareness of the changes in their abilities.[6]

Return to Case Examples: To illustrate how the program is actually carried out, it may be useful to return to the three patients described initially and to note their patterns of abilities and the sorts of work tasks they were assigned to make the most of their assets and minimize or improve weak areas. The first patient, Anne, had problems with sudden sleep onset and low frustration tolerance. She also had relatively severe visual deficits, tended to give up at the first sign of difficulty, and was easily sidetracked. Anne's strengths included her responsiveness to positive feedback and her willingness to attempt new tasks. To minimize the degree to which her sleepiness interfered with work performance, Anne was assigned tasks which were active in nature, requiring her for the most part to be going from place to place in the hospital rather than remaining in one spot and, inevitably, falling asleep. Anne's two primary work assignments involved collecting paper from various offices for a paper recycling project and watering the plants throughout the hospital. These tasks were difficult for Anne because she was easily distracted by opportunities for social interaction and also because her visual limitations made finding things difficult at times. However, Anne found it easy to stay awake and was very motivated because she could appropriately greet many people. In addition, these tasks were similar each day, enabling Anne to establish a visual scanning routine which minimized the effects of her deficit in this area. When the Jacobs was administered at a later time, it showed that while Anne compensated well for visual loss on her daily tasks, she did not generalize her compensatory strategies to the novel tasks on the Jacobs, indicating the need for changes in her routine to facilitate generalization (e.g., Gobble & Pfahl, 1985).

The second patient, Joey, had a number of good physical skills and was willing and motivated to work on interesting tasks for relatively long periods of time. However, his motor planning, sequencing, decision making, and problem solving skills were poor. When

Joey came to a difficult section of a task, he did not become frustrated and angry, as Anne did, but rather just stopped working and passively waited until directed what to do next. In addition, his very poor short term memory made it difficult for Joey to learn new tasks or adapt to new people and his disorientation made punctuality a real problem. To help him get to work on time, Joey was given a point card with his schedule on it and opportunities for earning points for timeliness. The work tasks chosen for him were ones which took advantage of his good motor skills but provided sufficient structure and cues so that Joey could perform the task. They were also repetitive enough that he could learn them. For example, when Joey was assigned to clean the workshop he was first assisted in making a list of each step in the process beginning with "get the broom from the corner." Over time, he was able to learn how to do a thorough job without specific instructions when given only the directive to clean the workroom.

Finally, Pamela, as mentioned previously, had fairly good clerical skills involving sorting, classifying, filing, sequencing, and mathematical calculation. Her main weaknesses were poor organizational skills, social inappropriateness (e.g., interruptions, poor listening skills), poor spatial memory, and limited task focus. While Joey was so disoriented that he was rarely on time, Pamela depended so heavily on her watch that her awareness of time distracted her from what she was working on. She was also initially unable to organize work materials even when she knew what needed to be done. Finally, Pamela had difficulty following directions and finding her way around the hospital. Pamela was given the tasks of stamping charge tickets and doing the "payroll" for herself and the other patients in prevocational training. The main focus of training was to increase her task focus and decrease her distractibility. To facilitate this initially, Pamela was asked to give her watch to the therapist when she arrived and let the therapist tell her when it was time to go. This strategy enabled Pamela to focus more on the task at hand, as did setting up the materials for her before she arrived. To work on improving her environmental mobility and social skills, Pamela was also asked to deliver charge tickets to the appropriate therapists. These tasks took advantage of Pamela's good math and clerical skills, improving her sense of worth and enabling her to tolerate the level of frustration associated with some of the more difficult aspects of her work.

In summary, the prevocational program at Cumberland Hospital is designed to help brain injured adolescents like these to develop appropriate work habits, attitudes, and skills necessary to work situations. Their problems are addressed in a worklike atmosphere to maintain motivation, facilitate generalization, and promote self esteem. However, the program is not designed to be the final step prior to a return or entry into competitive work. Currently, most of the patients go on to other work training programs (both outpatient and inpatient) following discharge from Cumberland in order to further develop their skills and then experience actual work trials in the community. For others, competitive work appears not to be a viable option and they are assisted in developing avocational interests and/ or participating in volunteer programs. The program has been well received thus far and continues to evolve.

REFERENCES

1. Adamovich BB, Henderson JA & Auerbach S. *Cognitive Rehabilitation of Closed Head Injured Patients*. San Diego: College Hill Press, 1985

2. Brooks DN (Ed.). *Closed head injury: Psychological, social, and family consequences*. New York: Oxford University Press, 1984

3. Lezak, MD. Living with the characterologically altered brain injured patient. *J Clin Psychiatry*, 29, 592-598, 1978

4. Rosenbaum M & Najenson R. Changes in life patterns and symptoms of low mood as reported by wives of severely brain-injured soldiers. *J Cons and Clin Psychology*, 44, 881-888, 1976

5. Jacobs K. *Occupational therapy: Work-related programs and assessments*. Boston: Little, Brown, & Co., 1985

6. Gobble EMR & Pfahl JC. Career development. In M. Ylvisaker (Ed.), *Head Injury Rehabilitation: Children and Adolescents (pp. 411-426)*. San Diego: College Hill Press, 1985

BOOK REVIEWS

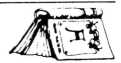

A GUIDE TO REHABILITATION. PM Deutsch & HW Sawyer. *Matthew Bender, 1275 Broadway, Albany, NY 12201, 1985, $80.00.*

A Guide to Rehabilitation is to rehabilitation counseling what Willard and Spackman's *Occupational Therapy* is to our profession. And similar to it, this book contains both the strengths and weaknesses of a comprehensive handbook for a profession that is noted for its diversity. The principle authors Deutsch and Sawyer aptly describe it as a guide for practitioners: it is an encyclopedia for the counselor describing assessment tools, evaluation formats, and professional techniques. Although I can not make knowledgable comment on all sections because of the book's breadth, I will review its overall quality and relevance to occupational therapy.

The book has two main sections. The first relates to vocational rehabilitation, an area traditionally associated with rehabilitation counseling. Chapters include evaluation and treatment of the client with a work history, assessing transferable skills, and vocational habilitation. Career information systems are also covered in a later chapter on computers. The second section of the book is an overview of rehabilitation of select disabilities, for example chronic pain, amputation, and back and neck injuries. These contain brief and superficial reviews of medical aspects of the disability, however, the comments on assessment and treatment offer current and very practical advice. In addition, four detailed case histories combining vocational and general rehabilitation information are presented. Unfortunately only one chapter addresses psychological disability and its treatment of the topic is inadequate.

161

One of the remarkable aspects of this book is the chapters on litigation including the professional as an expert witness, courtroom procedures and techniques, and determination of economic loss. The therapist involved in vocational rehabilitation or assessment for legal purposes will find these of use. The chapter on computer application in rehabilitation is also excellent, containing information on psychological and vocational assessment software. Both of these topics are covered in unusual detail for the handbook and include extensive bibliographies and resource lists. Another strength of this book is the economic orientation taken in the specific disability chapters. These include detailing the average costs of treatments and appliances and estimations of overall cost of recovery for specific disabilities. I think the realities of the economics of disability have not yet been adequately addressed in occupational therapy and this book provides a good example of how it can be.

The format of the book is also notable. Deutsch and Sawyer have truly adopted the "handbook" style of presentation of material making ample use of comparative tables and charts to summarize such information as averge periods of disability for head injuries, cost of orthoses, and types of intellectual assessment. The notion of "handbook" is also evident in the screw mount binding of the book. The authors intend to update this book with information that could be easily inserted much like notes into a binder. I hope that they are able to make good this promise as it would help keep the practitioner current in the rapidly changing field of rehabilitation.

The weakness inherent in comprehensive handbooks is that in illustrating the breadth of the field, topics are not covered in depth. Although the references for each chapter in this book are appropriate and in the main up to date, they are disappointingly sparse. Importantly, theoretical background has been sacrificed for detailed technical information in this book, leaving the impression of a "cook book" approach to rehabilitation. One chapter that is particularly weak is psychosocial adaptation, an important area in both counseling and occupational therapy. Moreover, the topics covered are those frequently encountered in counseling, excluding areas commonly dealt with by therapists for example pediatrics and gerontology.

Despite its problems I recommend this book as a reference for some therapists, specifically those in vocational rehabilitation, private practice, and those dealing with litigation. These areas of expanding practice in occupational therapy could benefit from adapting or borrowing knowledge from rehabilitation counseling. *A Guide to Rehabilitation* is also of use to educators because of the extensive case histories involved. And as a resource for such specific information as addresses for obtaining cognitive retraining material, and prevalence and incidence of extremity amputation it is invaluable. But at $75.00 this is not a book everyone ought to purchase. Moreover, despite the authors claims that this is relevant to all professionals, it is too narrowly focused to be used as a general reference in occupational therapy.

Laura Harvey Krefting, MA, OT(C)

VOCATIONAL REHABILITATION OF THE INJURED WORK-ER. LL Deneen & TA Hessellund. *Rehabilitation Publications, PO Box 23606, San Francisco, CA 94122, 1981, 172 pp, $24.75.*

Vocational Rehabilitation of the Injured Worker could easily serve as a textbook for a new breed of private vocational rehabilitation counselors. The forward is written by Thomas Porter, Professor of Rehabilitation and Special Education at Auburn University in Alabama. He writes that the text will attract the maverick, the problem solver who feels it necessary to produce credible results in assisting the injured worker to achieve work productivity.

Deneen and Hessellund write from a broad and extensive base of practical experience. Readers with academic preparation and professional skill in vocational rehabilitation counseling will find it an excellent guide for entering private practice.

The new role of the rehabilitation counselor entering this private practice arena includes accountability as representative, counsel, and intermediary to employer, physician, lawyer, and insurance claims agent. His former role as client advocate expands to assisting the client in dealing with all of the systems involved with the worker's compensation process. The private counselor deals with the real world of work; he is now a business person.

Specific chapters on Worker's Compensation law and requirements include a good description of a qualified injured worker, perceptive and helpful guidelines for identification of needs and procedures necessary for successful communication in processing client needs. Job analysis is an essential skill of the rehabilitation counselor. It identifies relevant, accurate and complete information about a particular job.

Chapters on accountability, ethical problems, and forensic implications also include external influences on the counselor and the need for professional objectivity within the legal climate in which he finds himself. Realistic personality and professional characteristics necessary to be successful in forensic vocational rehabilitation are given. Skills of vocational diagnosis, vocational exploration and rehabilitation planning, client motivation, interpersonal and job seeking skills are client oriented. Case histories support the given techology.

Deneen and Hessellund have done extensive counseling work, lecturing and research in California. Statistics and very descriptive definitions of agency roles and functions are those of California. However, the information, trends and concepts are nationally meaningful.

A bonus for the new private rehabilitation counselor is the chapter on "hidden agendas" which include biases, attitudes, hopes, fears, and the counselor's psychological climate; factors which are seldom confronted but can be used advantageously by the counselor.

Deneen and Hessellund describe the injured worker vocational rehabilitation client to the counselor, "your clients are those workers whose injuries have left them with a residual impairment, making it impossible for them to return to their former jobs or to seek work in allied fields. The nature of their disability prevents them from performing in their former jobs with industrially acceptable skill and speed. These are the workers who become candidates for vocational rehabilitation and eventually your clients." (Vocational Rehabilitation for the Industrially Injured, Deneen & Hessellund, 1981, p. 16-17).

The authors have carefully defined a different category of vocational rehabilitation clients. These were workers used to gainful employment. They desire to be productive, receive familiar wages, and work benefits. They are not the traditional vocational rehabilitation client, the chronically disabled client in the social climate. They are not the temporarily disabled injured worker returning to jobs after a short term of recuperation with competent medical help.

The book ends on an encouraging, hopeful note, supported by

success ratios. Counseled injured worker clients find work at 92-94 percent of former earning capacity.

Occupational therapists interested in work evaluation are urged to read and digest this text. Much more is involved here than just a good text for private vocational rehabilitation counselors, or an excellent procedure format for vocational rehabilitation of the injured worker.

The occupational therapist work evaluator also invests in training and work evaluator skills in direct service to the injured worker, physician, lawyer, employer and insurance intermediary. Mechanisms of counseling, testing, job analysis, work sampling, forensic intervention, etc., will appear identical to a casual or unskilled reader.

Occupational therapists interested in forensic, private work evaluation of the injured worker must read this book. It brings us into a new arena for rehabilitation of the injured worker.

Edwinna Marshall, MA, OTR

PATHWAYS TO EMPLOYMENT FOR ADULTS WITH DEVELOPMENTAL DISABILITIES. WE Kiernan and JA Stark (Eds). *Paul H. Brookes Publishing Co., PO Box 10624, Baltimore, MD 21285-0624, 1986, 321 pp, $39.95.*

The forty-three contributors to this text are major authorities in the area of developmental disabilities. Recognizing the paucity of available data in this field, the editors determined to offer a comprehensive plan for meeting the social, vocational and residential needs of persons with handicaps for whom it is vital to prepare for, secure, and hold a job.

A model is presented that focuses on the capacities of a disability and the educational transition to the adult world of work. The chief concern is to facilitate and improve the provision of services for the majority of young people with developmental disabilities who are not making a successful transition from special education programs to the community because of inadequate employment opportunities. It is reported that isolated environments, whether institutions, workshops or residential settings do not provide an appropriate approach to the needs for interaction with non-disabled persons.

The authors agree that the service system for the developmentally disabled adult often provides limited options for housing, work, and leisure. Most support programs promote dependency and discourage employment. However, they say there are trends operating in society today which are having a favorable impact on developmentally disabled citizens, giving them opportunities for movement within the system and active participation in the decision making process that will affect their training and work-related experiences.

The book presents discussions on the functional definitions of developmental disabilities, on public service programs, supported training vs. employment alternatives, contemporary management changes for special employees, medical care needs, and residential options. It provides a framework of choices for work environments and employment methods that should be available in a real work setting for the purpose of increasing productivity, expanding self-sufficiency and allowing the individual with a developmental disability to be an asset to society, not an economic liability.

Training strategies, research efforts, and evaluation practices are examined to show that there are both successful vocational transition programs integrated with community-based employment opportunities for special education students, and supported work programs which demonstrate that the actual work locale is essential in preparing adults with developmental disabilities to enter competitive employment outside the workshop. New designs offer habilitation components for the ongoing support of these adults while training in the regular work environment as well as responding to needs outside the workplace.

The writers interweave their respective views on the major issues related to substantial work for individuals with developmental disabilities. They challenge involved personnel to work together to ensure these persons the appropriate training methods that will satisfy the needs they face in their adult years.

This book is extremely encouraging to those who have chosen to work on behalf of adults with developmental disabilities. It is comprehensive and absorbs the reader's attention as the factors associated with the provision of effective services are analyzed and new models of practice recommended. It is of concern that the text is addressed to special educators, vocational counselors, and psychologists, omitting reference to other professionals whose holistic philosophies equip them to make significant contributions to the assessment and training of persons with developmental disabilities. Occupational therapists in this field will find invaluable information on changing patterns, and assistance on how to structure current and future delivery systems. Therapists play an integral part in the team approach, laying a foundation that ensures disabled adults successful experiences as they undergo the stressful changes of leaving school and entering the world of work.

Helen E. Lowe, OTR

OCCUPATIONAL THERAPY ASSISTANT: A PRIMER. H Hirama. *Chess Publications, Inc., 232 East University Parkway, Baltimore, MD 21218, 1986, 267 pp, softcover, $18.95.*

THE CERTIFIED OCCUPATIONAL THERAPY ASSISTANT: ROLES AND RESPONSIBILITIES. SE Ryan (Ed). *Slack Incorporated, 6900 Grove Ave., Thorofare, NJ 08086, 1986, 495 pp, hardcover, $29.50.*

The emergence in 1986 of two textbooks written for and about occupational therapy assistants has provided validation of the certified occupational therapy assistant (COTA) as an integral member of the profession of occupational therapy. Although each book represents a vastly different style, each provides relevant and current information regarding the role and broad scope of practice of the COTA.

Dr. Hirama's primer meets the challenge well. It is truly "an elementary textbook—a book which covers the basic elements of any subject."[1] The subject of the occupational therapy assistant is clearly, concisely and factually presented in a well-organized and easily readable format. The book includes a detailed Table of Contents which outlines four major sections: Overview of Occupational

---

[1]*The American Heritage Dictionary of the English Language.* Boston: American Heritage Publishing Co. 1975

Therapy; General Occupational Therapy Assistant Skills, i.e., reports and records, evaluation, treatment planning; Specific Occupational Therapy Assistant Skills, i.e., therapeutic use of self, therapeutic exercise and equipment, splinting; Patient Conditions, i.e., developmental disabilities, cerebral palsy, psychiatry.

Each of the twenty three chapters includes well-stated learning objectives, chapter summary, review questions, additional learning activities, references and a suggested reading, listening and audiovisual list. The glossary is complete and proves to be an important adjunct to the text. The book's organization makes it a useful text for students, practicing COTAs and OTRs and educators. The text can be most effectively used during an orientation to occupational therapy course, with a need for supplementation in advanced classes.

Ms. Ryan has edited a textbook which is rich in contributions from experts in various specialty areas. Many of the chapters are co-written by a COTA/OTR team which is illustrative of the existing and potential working relationships between the COTA and OTR. The comprehensive nature of the book provides the reader with the opportunity to use the detailed Table of Contents for easy reference. As with the Hirama text, the Ryan text is clearly divided into major sections. The first section includes Historical Perspectives and the COTA: A Chronological Review; the second section, Core Knowledge, i.e., theoretical frameworks and approaches, human development; the third section covers Intervention Strategies, i.e., the child with cerebral palsy, the depressed adolescent, the adult stroke patient; the fourth section addresses Models of Practice, i.e., the role of the OTR and COTA in hospice care, the role of the COTA as an activities director; the fifth section includes Concepts of Practice – a very innovative section which incorporates information on the use of contemporary media, i.e., video recording, computers, small electronic devices; and the final section covers Contemporary Issues and Trends, i.e., intraprofessional relationships and socialization, the maturation process and principles of occupational therapy ethics.

The text does not include a glossary, an obvious omission in light of the sophisticated vocabulary throughout the book. However, the text contains an excellent collection of appendices. It is particularly strengthened by the use of case histories to illustrate theoretical information, and the examples of documentation provide a pragmatic aspect to the text.

Ms. Ryan's book can be used as the major text throughout the COTA curriculum and is also an excellent reference for practicing COTAs and OTRs. I was disappointed, however, with the overly specific nature of the section which outlines intervention strategies. For example, the chapters which describe the treatment of psychiatric disorders are limited. The omission of discussion regarding the depressed adult, chemically dependent adult or schizophrenic adult creates a section which does not consider the developmental continuum.

Each book represents a wealth of information previously available only through meticulous piecing together of published and non-published articles, chapter excerpts and lecture notes. As an educator I find that the availability of these excellent texts will certainly provide the professional community with current and valuable information. The role of the COTA has finally been recognized and well documented.

Karen Vermeul Taback, EdD, OTR

THE HAND: FUNDAMENTALS OF THERAPY. J Boscheinen-Morrin, V Davey, WB Conolly. *Butterworth Publishers, Borough Green, Seven Oaks, Kent TN 15 8PH England (US source: 80 Montvale Ave., Stoneham, MA 02180), 225 pp, $14.95(US).*

The Hand: Fundamentals of Therapy provides an easy-to-use first level reference and treatment guide for hand care. This complete and concise text gives the physician or therapist reader a good anatomical kinesiological and physiological background for over eleven categories of hand afflictions. The types of hand injuries and diseases reveiwed are those commonly found in the hand clinic of a general hospital.

To aid the process of examination the specific symptoms, signs and course of each hand problem is clearly identified. Photographs and diagrams are used frequently to supplement the text and to provide a quick recall of relevant physical signs. The recommended treatment course is provided with its possible problems and complications. The descriptions include the technical details when appropriate to either perform or to construct required intervention. The medical and therapeutic information is up to date and well referenced.

The authors are to be commended on the precision with which they prioritize and focus on the many hand care problems in such a concise manner. This small book with its accurate, rich detail is very useful clinically for interning physicians and therapists as well as for general practitioners. No words are wasted and no words are minced, and yet unlike other hand care references, it is very complete. Unfortunately, it is just a bit too tall to fit conveniently in a laboratory coat pocket, where it belongs!

Jane Bear-Lehman, MS, OTR, OT(C)

OCCUPATIONAL THERAPY IN THE TREATMENT OF ADULT HEMIPLEGIA. O Eggers. *Aspen Systems Corporation, 1600 Research Blvd., Rockville, MD 20850, 1984, 147 pp, $15.00.*

This little book is wonderful if your intent is to incorporate Bobath Principles into occupational therapy treatment with stroke patients. The author is an occupational therapist from Basel, Switzerland and the book was originally published as *Ergotherapiebei Hemiplegie*, 2nd edition, 1982. This edition was translated by an occupational therapist in London.

The uniqueness of the book is that the major focus is on an extensive array of creative, practical ideas for treatment with patients with hemiplegia. Treatment suggestions are given for specific problems and all lie within the occupational therapy realm of practical application and functional activity. All the treatment suggestions incorporate Bobath principles, i.e., normalizing tone, working for symmetry, avoiding associated reactions, facilitation of normal movements. The many illustrations reinforce the text and are so graphic that it is easy to see how positioning is done and how activities can be set up and adapted as well as to see what they are designed to accomplish.

Three major chapters give treatment aims and suggestions for: general motor problems, e.g., neglect of the hemiplegic side; different stages of recovery of the arm and hand, e.g., stage 1-no function in arm and hand; and sensory deficits. Suggestions include: total body positioning; bilateral, bimanual and unilateral activities utilizing games, puzzles, crafts and ADL. Activities can be positioned in a variety of planes and adapted to meet individual needs. There are extensive suggestions for treatment of sensory deficits combined with motor training using a variety of shapes, textures and positions incorporated into activities.

In addition, there is an excellent chapter on treatment media with many ideas of appropriate furniture, suitable techniques to use with crafts and games, and ideas on how to adapt them to create new ones. Areas that are covered, but in less detail, include: Assessment of motor function, ideas for bilateral group activities, and ways to introduce "controlled" one handed training without ignoring the affected side. There is also an introduction to Bobath principles which reinforces the need to refer to Berta Bobath references for more detail on specific techniques.

Throughout the book there is an emphasis on the need to look at a patient as an individual and to design activities that suit him, to be ready to modify and adapt the activity as well as to address the needs of the whole person including social, psychological, and perceptual. There are so many concrete treatment suggestions throughout the book that it can be used very effectively as a resource, to refer to as new patients and problems emerge. Principles behind each activity are stressed so much that the ideas can be used as a spring board to create new activities to meet specific needs.

Edith Gillespie, MEd, OTR

TEST OF VISUAL-PERCEPTUAL SKILLS. MF Gardner. *JB Preston (Ed and Publisher), PO Box 33548, Seattle, WA 98133 (order from: Children's Hospital of San Francisco, Publications Department, OPR-110, PO Box 3805, San Francisco, CA 94119), 1982, $55.00.*

The *Test of Visual-Perceptual Skills* (TVPS) (Nonmotor) was published by Morrison F. Gardner of Children's Hospital, San Francisco in 1982. It was designed to measure seven distinct areas of a child's visual-perceptual skills. These areas are visual discrimination, visual memory, visual-spatial relationships, visual form constancy, visual sequential memory, visual figure ground and visual closure.

Each of the seven subtests contain 16 items and are arranged in order of difficulty with a ceiling for each subtest. The test was standardized on approximately 1,200 children residing within the San Francisco Bay Area. The children ranged in age from 4 years through 12 years, 11 months. No significant differences were found in sex.

A probability sampling technique was used to approximate the range and level of ability of children in the U.S. population. Reliability studies exhibited adequate reliability for each subtest and the test as a whole for each age level. Lower internal consistency was found with older children on some subtests where a ceiling effect was evident. No test retest reliability was conducted.

Content, item, diagnostic, criterion-related and predictive validity was examined during the development of the test. The TVPS validity studies lent support that the tests identify deficits in visual perception.

Testing time varies from 7 to 15 minutes depending on the chronological age and ability of the child. The test is extremely easy to administer. The author states that no advanced training or education is required, however, the TVPS should be administered by professionals who are familiar with testing procedures. This reviewer feels that test administration is not as precise as some of the Sensory Integration and Praxis Tests by A. Jean Ayres, OTR, PhD.

Scoring is simple and takes approximately 5 minutes. Test results have been converted into perceptual ages, scaled scores and percentiles for each subtest and median perceptual ages for the combined scores of the seven subtests.

The author feels that a meaningful interpretation for individuals

13 years old through adult can be made. TVPS performance levels off toward early adolescence and he feels that it is reasonable to expect that normal individuals age 13 or older would perform within the same statistical limits as the oldest children in the standardization sample. This reviewer thinks that therapists should exercise caution when using standard scores with adults. Visual form and space perception is thought to continue to develop until age 15 years. This reviewer feels that it would be inappropriate to use age equivalent scores for adults. Scaled scores could be used to report progress in various subtests.

Visual perceptual forms used in the test are felt to be non-language based as well as culturally unbiased which adds to the advantages of the test.

Because of its nonmotor component, this reviewer feels that this would be a good test to evaluate visual perception in those individuals that have a neuromuscular disorder such as cerebral palsy. Nonspeech individuals could easily be evaluated and even switch devices could be used to indicate choices if the individual was unable to point to the correct picture. Visual form and space perception could be evaluated in children with developmental dyspraxia which influences paper and pencil tasks.

In summary, this test could be used by occupational therapists to evaluate various areas of visual form and space perception, especially when a motor component might influence the outcome.

Dottie M. Ecker, MA, OTR, FAOTA

MEALTIMES FOR PERSONS WITH SEVERE HANDICAPS. R Perske, A Clifton, BM McLean, and JI Stein. *Paul H. Brookes Publishing Co., PO Box 10624, Baltimore, MD 21285-0624, 1986, 136 pp, $16.95.*

This book is a revised edition of the original published in 1977. It is a compilation of many authors. Each contributor briefly discusses different aspects of mealtimes with severely handicapped individuals. Among the authors are educators, program administrators, occupational therapists, parents and severely handicapped people themselves. The purpose of the book is to present, in easily readable terms, various views on this topic and this purpose is well accomplished. The editors were spurred on in this effort by various experiences in institutions or schools where they saw individuals being fed lying down, being bird fed, being fed too rapidly or being fed in very undesirable atmospheres.

Because of having numerous contributors with different ideas the book does contain some conflicting information but this seems well in line with the reality of having various opinions. This reviewer feels the book has much excellent information and highly recommends it for therapists working with severely handicapped individuals. It is also an excellent book for parents and caretakers in terms of alerting them to the sensitivities of the individual and the importance of the mealtime experience. Administrators of institutions can also benefit from this text not just to get ideas about mealtimes but to get the general sensitivity that they need in order to run the institution's feeding programs in a manner that encourges the highest level of developmental progress possible.

The various chapters vary greatly from straightforward factual information regarding dental care, or reflexes and how they interfere with feeding, to those outlining thoughts and feelings of aides and/or parents involved in mealtime programs. As an occupational therapist, I feel the book really hits home with some of the mealtime problems that often occur or bad habits that caretakers fall into when feeding profoundly handicapped individuals. Several of the chapters talk about what one author calls the ''hen party'' syndrome where the aides or technicians talk about the soap operas or what they did the night before while rapidly feeding two or three children. Many of the contributors point out the importance of direct conversation to the child during the meal and the potential for improving social and communication skills at mealtimes. Many helpful suggestions are made as to set-up of dining areas as well as ways to clue the child by time, place, or routine as to when eating is about to occur.

Chapters written by severely handicapped people themselves are highlights. One written by Dr. Edward Roberts details how he as a young polio survivor was fed in the hospital. We are lucky that he can put into words his unhappiness with being forced to eat things at a rate determined by somebody else and forced to eat foods selected by somebody else. He reinforces the need for caregivers to try to read the individual's nonverbal communication as to what he or she does not like. The chapter written by a severely involved cerebral palsy man, Fred Markham, talks about the experience of eating out. He talks about how important it is for him to explain to someone who is going out with him for the first time that he does need a great deal of help in order to eat. He also talks about his need to explain to companions that people will and do stare at him while he is being fed by another in a restaurant. But he also explains the need that he has as a human being to be able to participate in the social enjoyment of dining out. One of the chapters written by a parent contains a recipe type program for an oral motor stimulation program for a young child. As long as this chapter is used for the purpose for which it was intended, and that was to illustrate a particular program and not provide a recipe for others, the information is valuable in showing how parents can devise innovative ways of fitting a demanding program into their daily schedule. The annotated bibliography has been updated and serves as a good resource as to what has been written in this area.

The book, even though it was first written and published in 1977 is still very needed today because as you go into institutions you still see so many of the problems that were cited as the instigation for the book. Although you may not see clients being fed in a lying down position as before, you still see many being fed too much too quickly and with no attempts at communication. Another thing that the book briefly mentions and unfortunately is being seen often today is the unnecessary use of gastrostomy tubes for feeding for ease and convenience of the caretakers rather than because the individual needs the gastrostomy.

There is much for occupational therapists to do in the field of feeding the severely handicapped. It is true that we cannot take over feeding each and every one of these individuals but we have to be there to monitor constantly how they are being fed and to provide continual inservice training. Some of the recent emphasis on ergonomics could easily be applied to institutional dining room settings. This book is an excellent and extremely readable resource for occupational therapists and anyone else working in the care of the severely handicapped who is truly interested in improving quality of life.

Betty Snow, OTR

PICTURE THIS—AN ILLUSTRATED GUIDE TO COMPLETE
DINNERS. S. Bachner. *Special Additions, Inc., Greenwich, CT,
1984, 72 pp, pbk., $24.95.*

Any occupational therapy clinic involved with training patients in
meal preparation would benefit from this well laid out guide.

The author, an occupational therapist, applies activity analysis to
the entire meal preparation process. The book's format encompasses preparation of a whole dinner, from salad to entree. Colorful, step by step illustrations take the reader through the process of
gathering ingredients and supplies as well as the actual preparation
of recipes. A kit of long handled measuring cups and spoons color
coded to the text may also be purchased.

This book's layout is well thought out and is visually very easy to
follow. Spiral binding makes it ideal for use in the kitchen. Simple
language has been used in giving instructions for each cooking step,
thus enabling patients with limited reading ability to follow readily.
The illustrations, provided by cartoonist and commercial artist,
Tony Di Preta, are wonderfully graphic and augment the text per-
fectly. They would provide appropriate action cues, independent of
the text, for non-English speaking patients or patients without ability to comprehend written materials.

A clear and logical breakdown of all the steps in the meal preparation process is provided. This makes the guide particularly helpful
to individuals new to cooking. The clinician would also find it a
beneficial tool for use with any patient needing help with work simplification and task organization.

Tasty recipes, an easy to use format, and clear language and illustrations make this book a sure-to-be-used treatment resource for the
occupational therapy clinic.

Ana Verran, OTR

AGRICULTURAL TOOLS, EQUIPMENT, MACHINERY AND BUILDINGS FOR FARMERS AND RANCHERS WITH PHYSICAL HANDICAPS, VOL. I. *Breaking New Ground, Purdue University, Department of Agricultural Engineering, West Lafayette, IN 47907, 1986, 200+ pp, $30.00.*

BREAKING NEW GROUND: A NEWSLETTER FOR FARMERS WITH PHYSICAL DISABILITIES. (Same source, write for information.)

Occupational therapists serving rural populations will wish to be alerted to two publications directed particularly to the problems of daily working encountered by farmers with physical handicaps. While I have not been able to examine the book/manual, the description of its content gives promise to very practical kinds of problem solving for farmers' individual difficulties resulting from amputation, paraplegia, stroke, etc.

The Newsletter (I had one copy of 12 pages) appears to be at least quarterly, was started under a grant from the Department of Education/National Institute for Handicapped Research and reflects both news of research and activities/seminars/conferences of interest to handicapped farmers as well as current, practical and timely information and illustrations about situations encountered by farmers with special problems. Subscription price, if any, is unknown.

This relatively new facility at Purdue is confronting needs which have heretofore not been well addressed in any concerted way. Even though many of us occupational therapists have heard of the difficulties and triumphs of individual farmer patients helped by our colleagues, this endeavor, combining farm knowhow with rehabilitation engineering, appears to be meeting a great need. My own first reaction was to wonder if any occupational therapists are involved on the research teams. It would certainly be the right place for one knowing farm activities and skilled and interested in solving technical ADL problems.

Do write for more information if you think you or some of your patients could find solutions there.

Florence S. Cromwell, Editor

MICROCOMPUTERS: CLINICAL APPLICATIONS. (Current Practice Series in Occupational Therapy, Vol. 1, No. 2). E Nelson Clark (Ed). *Slack Incorporated, 6900 Grove Rd., Thorofare, NJ 08086, 1986, 72 pp, $14.50.*

This book has been designed as an introductory guide for occupational therapists considering the use of a computer in their practice. The six brief chapters cover topics related to business and treatment use of the computer. An appendix provides a listing of manufacturers and distributors of software and equipment to adapt the computer for disabled individuals.

The chapters are written in language which would be understood by someone without any prior computer experience. The book would have been improved as a "one-stop" source of beginning microcomputer knowledge if pictures of microcomputers and a glossary of computer terminology were included. The chapters on the use of the computer in visual perceptual and typing training are written at a very basic level. The chapter on alternative input systems is written at a higher level and would have been improved by a brief glossary of terms.

The book appears to be directd to the therapist who works in a traditional physical disabilities institutional setting. The chapter on how to justify the capital purchase of a microcomputer would be very helpful to a therapist in this setting. Therapists in private practice may find the chapters on treatment applications helpful and the appendix very useful in locating software for their practices.

In summary, *Microcomputers: Clinical Applications* is a good beginning review book for occupational therapists considering the purchase of a microcomputer.

Suzanne McLean, OTR

UNDERSTANDING THE PROSPECTIVE PAYMENT SYSTEM: A BUSINESS PERSPECTIVE. CM Baum and A Luebben. *Slack Incorporated, 6900 Grove Rd., Thorofare, NJ 08086, 1986, 100 pp, $11.50.*

This Book provides an impressive and comprehensive discussion of the prospective payment system. The book's purpose, as defined in the introduction, is to assist clinicians in understanding the prospective payment system and to provide management strategies to survive within the system.

Chapter 1 concentrates on providing the historical perspective leading up to the implementation of diagnostic related groups (DRGs).

Chapter 2 focuses on how to function under the prospective payment system. Measures are suggested whereby costs can be contained and growth can be accomplished.

Chapter 3 is devoted to addressing specialized skills necessary for the management of patients, programs, and resources. A stimulating self assessment tool is included, and brings the reader to the final chapter on innovative programming and managing change.

Finally, a resource guide is provided.

Baum and Luebben have written a valuable guide for occupational therapists who continue to practice within the ever changing health care system.

Julie Shuer, MA, OTR